A Basic Introduction to Speech Perception

Jack Ryalls, Ph.D.

University of Central Florida
Orlando, Florida

SINGULAR PUBLISHING GROUP, INC.

SAN DIEGO · LONDON

Singular Publishing Group, Inc.
401 West A Street, Suite 325
San Diego, California 92101-7904

19 Compton Terrace
London, N1 2UN, UK

Typeset in 11/13 Melior by So Cal Graphics
Printed in the United States of America by McNaughton & Gunn

Library of Congress Cataloging-in-Publication Data
Ryalls, Jack.
    A basic introduction to speech perception / Jack Ryalls.
      p.   cm. — (The speech science series)
    Includes bibliographical references and index.
    ISBN 1-56593-617-5
    1. Speech perception. I. Title. II. Series.
BF463.S64R83   1996
  152.1'5—dc20
                                            96–7531
                                                  CIP

Contents

Foreword

The study of speech perception has flourished in the last half of this century and now embraces an exciting and expanding literature. Contributors to this literature come from many specialities, including sensory and cognitive psychology, psycholinguistics, communication engineering, artificial intelligence, audiology, and speech-language pathology. Curiously, almost no books of introductory level have been written to open this field to a wider audience. As a consequence, speech perception often has occupied a marginal position in university and college curricula. Despite the central importance of speech perception to an understanding of communicative processes and disorders, basic information on this field is not readily available to students in speech pathology, audiology, psychology, or related fields. Jack Ryalls' *A Basic Introduction to Speech Perception* is a welcome text that will introduce students to experiments, concepts, and theories in the field of speech perception. The book is written with a comfortable and easy style that is well matched to the systematic coverage of basic information on how humans perceive speech. It is a gateway to a vigorous and important area of research on the human faculty of communication.

Ray D. Kent, Ph.D.

Preface

A few years ago, when I was scouting about for teaching materials for an undergraduate course I was asked to teach on speech perception, I made a rather startling discovery. While there are several very good texts on speech production, speech acoustics, and even some excellent chapters here and there on speech perception, I could not find a single textbook on speech perception!

This book is meant to fill this gap. It is intended, first of all, to provide undergraduate students with a basic introduction to speech perception. Many of the students who use this text may be undergraduate majors in either speech-language pathology or audiology. But this text might also be used in basic courses in linguistics or psychology. Although directed primarily to the undergraduate reader, it is also intended to serve as a basic introduction for the graduate student who has never previously studied speech perception. The text can be supplemented for a graduate course with the suggestions for further reading at the end of each chapter.

The book is written with the uninitiated reader in mind. It will be accessible to anyone who wants to find out more about speech perception, no matter what his or her background. It could, for example, be useful for parents trying to comprehend their own child's problem understanding speech. It might also serve those who want to understand the loss of hearing for speech that often occurs with advancing age. It should also be useful for speech-language pathologists or audiologists in the clinical setting who want to refresh their understanding of speech perception or wish to better inform a client or concerned parent.

Since this text is meant for such a broad audience, it is written in as simple, nontechnical language as possible. It is also limited to basic information on speech perception. At the end of each chapter the reader is directed to other material where more detailed information can be found. Many research articles are also referenced in the text and in the bibliography at the end, where the interested reader can turn for more complete information and additional references.

Most of this text was written while I was on sabbatical from the University of Montreal. I would like to thank my former department chairman, Dr. Yves Joanette, and other members of the Ecole d'orthophonie et d'audiologie at the University of Montreal for their support of my sabbatical—especially Dr. Guylaine Le Dorze and Dr. Jean-Pierre Gagné who read and made comments on earlier drafts. I would also like to thank the School of Human Communication Sciences and Disorders at McGill University for hosting me during my sabbatical, especially professor emeritus Don Doehring, who lent me use of his inspiring office, and to Dr. Shari Baum, who acted as chair during my stay at McGill. Dr. Linda Polka, also at McGill, prepared the auditory stimuli which produced Figure 5–4. She also read and made many useful suggestions on the chapters on infant perception and development.

The Fonds de la Recherche en Santé Médicale provided a grant during the sabbatical. I would like to extend my warm appreciation to Christine Brassard who dug up many references and provided much of the graphic work in this text. Additional graphic work, initially used for my undergraduate course in Speech and Hearing Science, was provided by Siglinde Quirk in the Graphics division of Instructional Resources at the University of Central Florida.

I would like to thank Dr. Tom Mullin at the University of Central Florida for his comments on earlier drafts and Heidi Hyche who located many of the references used in the last chapter.

Thanks go to Marie Linvill and to Angie Singh at Singular Publishing Group for their assistance, patience, and persistence; and especially to Professor Ray Kent, Singular's Speech Science Series Editor, for his initial encouragement and the insightful comments and suggestions he has made along the way, which have resulted in a much improved text.

I would also to thank my mentors Dr. Philip Lieberman and Dr. Sheila Blumstein at the Department of Cognitive and Linguistic Sciences at Brown University. Most of what I know about speech perception I first learned from them, and hopefully this text has benefited from their fine teaching and their exemplary research and mentorship.

Finally, I would like to thank the students who have sat through my courses (at Indiana University, the University of Montreal, and the University of Central Florida) and helped me to better understand speech perception by asking just the right questions. The old adage "the best way to learn about something is to have to teach it!" could not be more appropriate than here. I have not forgotten that without students I would not have written this book in the first place.

CHAPTER

1

The Sounds of Speech

LEARNING OBJECTIVES

The purpose of this chapter is to make the reader aware of some of the special properties of human speech. Speech is produced with the goal of perception on the part of a listener.

Vowel sounds are then discussed in detail, including some of their particular unique acoustic properties. The difference between voiced and voiceless sounds is considered as well as the source-filter theory of speech production. The vowel sounds are presented in terms of their articulation properties or features. The goal is to familiarize the reader with some of the particular acoustic properties of vowels in order to better understand the listener's perception of them.

A discussion of consonant sounds follows. The consonants are treated in terms of their various types, and their sound features are specified. Again, the goal is to make the reader aware of the distinguishing sound properties of vowels in order to appreciate the perception of consonants.

Human speech is not made up of just any old sounds, although you might get this impression when first listening to a foreign language. If there is anything we have learned from the past 50 years of research on speech it is just how special and well-suited speech is to the rapid and reliable transmission of information.

We'll see that in serving this twofold requirement of being both *rapid* and *reliable*, speech is a highly specialized form of sound. Just to underscore its rapidity, it has been estimated that speech can be understood at rates approaching *10 times faster than any other code* (Liberman, Cooper, Shankweiler & Studdert-Kennedy, 1967). As for reliability, it has been estimated that speech is approximately 50% redundant—that is, half of the information is transmitted in more than one manner. An example of redundancy in a written text is the shorthand notes that consist of leaving out many of the vowel letters—u cn stll smtms ndrstnd wrttn txts wth th vwls mssng.

We understand spoken words not only through their sounds, but through their meanings as well. In addition to the acoustic signal, we also use information such as whether or not a particular sequence of sounds is a word of English, as well as how our understanding of a word or sentence fits in with our "real world" knowledge.

An important principle for understanding human speech is that speech production is organized with speech perception in mind. That is, the speech sounds (or phonemes) of the world's languages have not been randomly selected. Rather, they were chosen because they are also sounds that are easily perceived by human beings. In other words, it is not just a chance occurrence that certain consonant sounds (such as p,t,k,b,d,g) and certain vowel sounds (such as ee, ah, oo) are found so often in different languages of the world.

Of course, the sounds used in a language must also be easy to produce. But if we think about it, a lot of sounds that we can easily produce are still not used in languages. Part of the reason they are not used is because they may not be well suited for perception. They are easy enough to produce, but perhaps much harder to hear reliably.

Before we can explore much about speech perception, it will be useful, and perhaps necessary for the uninitiated reader, to consider some of the basic facts about speech sounds. Therefore, we'll first consider some basic information about how speech is produced and its special acoustic nature, before we consider how it is perceived. We need to have at least some basic understanding of the special way in which speech is produced in order to make better sense of the way it is perceived. This is an important fact about speech, although perhaps deceptively obvious: **Speech is produced by a speaker in order to be understood by a listener.** We speak not just to hear ourselves, but rather to relay a specific message.

This may seem ridiculously simple and patently obvious. Yet it is important to constantly remain aware of this intimate relationship between the production and perception of human speech. It is all too easy to concentrate our attention on the more obvious and visible component of speech—the speech producer, the speaker. But a speech act has not occurred until speech is also understood by a listener.

The largely invisible and deceptively effortless process on the part of the listener in perceiving speech turns out to be incredibly complex. It is as if mother nature has hidden some of the complexity of the process in order to allow us to concentrate on our goal of making sense out of speech. This is fortunate, because if we had to consciously pay attention to all the processes involved in perceiving speech sounds, we probably wouldn't have the time to understand much of what was actually being said, before it had already faded away.

We usually overlook the inherently ephemeral nature of speech. Speech sounds only remain suspended in the air for a few brief moments. If we aren't quick to grab for meaning, speech may disappear from the sound environment without a trace.

The emphasis on production of speech is probably because this is the more visible end of speech—we can see our lips and feel our tongue move. Even though they are not visible, we can feel the vibration of our vocals folds if we place our fingers on our throats as we speak. But we don't see phonemes in the air, and we certainly don't have much visible sign that speech is being perceived. Neither ears nor brains give much outward sign of their activity. Sometimes the only evidence of speech perception we have may be the confused look on people's faces when they have *not* understood what was said.

So tightly linked are speech production and its perception, that one theory of speech perception that will be considered at a later point (the so-called *motor theory* of speech perception) is based on this association. This theory basically proposes that speech perception is based on its production. Whether this theory is actually the best account of speech perception or not, does not alter the importance of this link between perception and production. Not only does speech employ sounds that are easily produced, these sounds must also be easily perceived—that is, one sound must be readily distinguished from another. Production limits the sounds of speech to those that can be produced by the human speech apparatus, and perception further limits these sounds to what humans can conveniently perceive. There is even evidence that human beings have undergone physical changes (i.e., in the angle between the oral and pharyngeal vocal tract) that enable them to produce certain speech sounds which are more perceptible (Lieberman, 1975).

Vowels

Let us consider some basic facts about speech sounds. First of all, as you already know, there are two main groups or classes of speech sounds: vowels and consonants. As we'll see, not only are they different in the manner in which they are produced, they seem to rely on somewhat different perceptual mechanisms as well. In some ways, vowels can be considered more basic or more prime speech sounds than consonants. Similar vowel sounds form both the basis for rhyme on which poetry is based, and tongue twisters. Speech errors are more likely to occur between words with similar vowels, even though the error is more likely to involve a consonant.

Among some of the almost magical properties sometimes associated with vowels are some people's claim that vowel sounds have an inherent natural color association—they "see" yellow for the "ee" vowel sound for example. This crossover between two sense modalities is termed *synesthesia*. Most people find the notion of such an association between color and sound a strange idea indeed. Yet it is intriguing to consider that there is some degree of consistency between vowel and color association across the many reports of this particular synesthetic experience. The association is far from being as random as one might expect (Ryalls, 1986).

From an articulatory standpoint, in a general manner, vowels are produced with the mouth open, whereas consonants are produced by closing the mouth, at least partially.

Vowels are almost always produced with the vocal folds vibrating. (They are called vocal folds these days instead of vocal cords, in recognition of the fact that they are attached along one edge and unlike a string or cord.) Only when vowels are whispered are they not voiced (i.e., produced with the vocal folds vibrating.) The vibrating vocal folds provide the source or sound basis for vowels, which is then modified or filtered by the particular shape of the mouth. The shape of the mouth is largely determined by movement of the tongue and the lips. This characterization of speech in terms of a sound source which is then modified by the vocal tract is known as the *source-filter theory of speech production*. The source is usually the sound emitted from the vibrating vocal folds, which is then filtered by the supralaryngeal vocal tract (supra = above, laryngeal = larynx or voice box). The *supralaryngeal vocal tract* refers to all of the throat above the vocal folds, including the oral cavity. Vowel sounds are voiced or produced with the vocal folds vibrating, except when whispered. In whispered vowels, the vocal folds still move but are not set into regular or full vibration.

Description of the Vowel Sounds of English

We can describe the particular vowels in terms of where the tongue is positioned in the oral cavity when they are spoken. The two main relevant dimensions of tongue movement are *up and down* and *front to back*. In the following discussion, slashes (//) will be used when we speak about a particular speech sound. Slashes denote that the symbols appearing between them refer to a phoneme—a basic speech sound, in this case, of the English language. The symbols are those of the International Phonetic Alphabet (IPA). They are similar to the symbols used in most dictionaries as guides to pronunciation. While a different sound can often be spelled several different ways, it will have a unique symbol in the phonetic alphabet. Although these symbols may not be familiar to you, unless you have taken a course in phonetics or have been taught phonetic transcription, each time they are used an example will also be given to indicate what sound is being discussed.

Starting from a "high front" vowel like /i/ (the vowel *ee* sound as in *pea*), in order of descending vowel height, we pass through the sound of /ɪ/ like in *pit*—the so-called short i; next is

/ɛ/ like in *pet*, /æ/ like in *pat*, and finally /ɑ/ like in *pot*. The back vowel series goes from /u/ to /ɔ/. (See Figure 1–1.) While this order generally seems accurate in terms of tongue placement, it should be borne in mind that some speakers do not seem to adhere to this exact pattern (Ladefoged, DeClerk, Lindau, & Papcun, 1972). In the center is a vowel which is neither high nor low, front nor back—the so called *central* or *neutral* vowel schwa, written /ʌ/ or /ə/ (depending on whether the syllable is stressed).

Vowels can also be considered as relatively slower to change, or more steady-state in nature. That is, even though they are relatively brief events, usually only several hundred milliseconds in duration, they are much slower to change than consonants. Consonants are characterized by a much more rapid and quickly changing articulation, and consequently the acoustic information that specifies them also changes very rapidly.

In addition to these so-called *pure* vowels, there are also vowels that change from one vowel to another called *diphthongs*. Diphthongs are heard in vowels like *bite, boy* or *cow*. You can hear how the vowel changes if you pronounce them to yourself very slowly. In typical American pronunciation, most vowels change at least slightly during their articulation. In other words, vowels are all somewhat "diphthongized" in American English. Vowels in a language like modern French are much less diphthong or pure (although they are diphthong in the French spoken in Canada, which has preserved the diphthong vowels of eighteenth century French). Changing vowel quality may be part of what typifies the sound of American English to the foreign ear, which some foreigners have described to sound like speaking while chewing gum.

Consonants

Description of Consonant Sounds

We need to describe the different types of consonant sounds in order to understand them better. In order to describe them, we'll make use of a classic framework that divides consonants along the lines of the differences in how they are spoken, and the con-

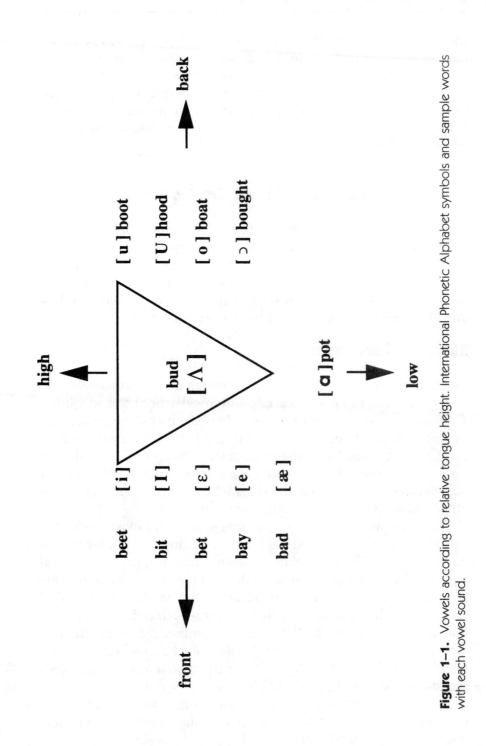

Figure 1–1. Vowels according to relative tongue height. International Phonetic Alphabet symbols and sample words with each vowel sound.

sequent differences in the resulting sound. It will be useful for the reader to refer to Figure 1–2 when necessary as we follow through the different groups of consonant sounds. Each distinction is treated in the order it appears in Figure 1–2 going from top to bottom. (Following this diagram in the opposite order from bottom to top then will guide the reader to basic characteristics of any particular consonant sound.)

Resonants Versus Occlusives

The first major distinction in consonant type is between *resonants* and *occlusives*. Occlusive consonants are produced by restricting or occluding the airstream as it makes its way up from the lungs, through the vocal folds, and out of the mouth. Resonant consonants are closer in nature to vowels because, like vowels, the vocal tract is not obstructed or occluded.

Resonant Consonants

There are two types of resonant consonants: *semivowels* and *nasals*. There are two types of semivowels: *liquids* and *glides*. The glides are the "sometime" vowels *y* and *w* that we all learned in elementary school (/j/ and /w/ in IPA). These sounds are similar to diphthongs since the articulators change position during their production. But semivowels are produced with greater approximation, or closure of the mouth, than diphthongs. The other semivowels are the liquids /r/ and /l/.

For the nasals, the mouth is somewhat more closed, and the lips are also more approximated, than during the production of vowel sounds. The soft palate or *velum*, which separates the oral and nasal cavities, is opened, and the airstream escapes out the nose, since the mouth is closed. The place where the mouth is shut the tightest—the place of maximal closure—determines the particular sound of each of the three nasal consonants. For /m/ the lips are squeezed together; therefore it is described as *bilabial* (bi = two, labial = lips). In /n/ the tongue tip is placed on the alveolar ridge—the mound on the gums just behind the teeth. For this reason, /n/ is known as the *alveolar* nasal. /ŋ/, the sound in the ending *ing* is described as *velar*, because the tongue is placed even further back, with the body of the tongue placed against the velum.

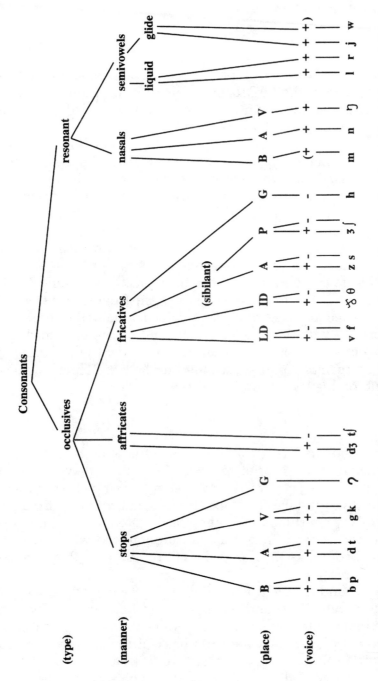

Figure 1–2. Consonants listed by articulatory features: B = bilabial, A = alveolar, V = velar, G = glottal, LD = labiodental, ID = interdental, P = palatal, + = voiced, – = voiceless. When written in parentheses, there are no contrasts by voicing. To obtain traditional descriptions, follow features from bottom to top of figure. For example, a /b/ is a "voiced, bilabial, stop."

Occlusive Consonants

Fricatives

There are three different types of occlusives, depending on the degree to which the airstream is obstructed. Occlusive consonants can be produced with or without the vocal folds vibrating, that is, with or without voicing.

In *fricative* consonants, the mouth is not shut and the airstream is not completely stopped. Rather, the airstream is merely directed through a narrowed space, which thus produces a distinctive sound or frication noise. A subgroup of fricatives, /s/, /z/, /θ/, and /ð/, are called *sibilants* because of their characteristic hissing sound. /s/ and /z/ are both produced with the tongue approximating the alveolar ridge, but the vocal folds are vibrating during /z/ and not during /s/.

There are two groups of nonsibilant fricatives. /f/ and /v/ are produced with the lower lip placed against the upper teeth, so they are called *labiodental*. /f/ is produced without the vocal folds vibrating, /v/ with them vibrating. /θ/ and /ð/ are produced with the tongue placed between the upper and lower teeth, so they are called *interdental*. /θ/, the last sound in the word *breath* is voiceless, but /ð/, the last sound in *breathe* is voiced.

Stops

Stop consonants are produced with the mouth completely closed, at least for a brief moment. Therefore, they are called stop consonants because the airstream is completely stopped. Like fricatives and nasals, stops are distinct because of their particular place of articulation—the place where the maximal oral constriction occurs. Since they are pronounced with a distinct explosive sound as they are released by the lips, they are also known as *plosives*.

For /p/ and /b/ the lips are tightly approximated, so they are termed *bilabial*. In /t/ and /d/ the constriction occurs where the tongue touches the alveolar ridge. And in /k/ and /g/ the place of maximal closure is where the back of the tongue is placed against the velum. Whereas /p/, /t/, and /k/ are produced without the activity of the vocal folds, their voiced equivalents /b/, /d/, and /g/ are produced with the vocal folds vibrating.

Actually, this description in terms of the mere presence or absence of voicing is somewhat of a simplification. Since the stop consonants have to be produced with at least a short vowel sound, and since vowels are generally produced with the vocal folds vibrating, the true difference between the so-called voiced and voiceless consonants turns out not to be a simple all or none distinction. Rather, the difference is one involving how much time occurs before the vocal folds begin to vibrate.

In the voiced stops, the vocal folds begin to vibrate very quickly after the mouth is opened and the consonant is "released" from the lips or tongue. In voiceless stops there is a greater delay after the consonant is released before the onset of vocal fold vibration. This difference in the onset of voicing is known as the *voice onset time*. (Usually this measure is performed only on the *periodic* portion of the voicing, that is, the portion where the vocal folds are vibrating in a regular pattern). We'll consider how particular changes in voice onset time influence perception in Chapter 5 on Categorical Perception.

Affricates

There are two affricates in English, /dʒ/, and /tʃ/ (Respectively the *g* sound in *beige*, and the *ch* sound in *change*.) Affricates begin like a stop, in that they start out with complete closure of the vocal tract like a stop consonant, but then they are changed or released into a fricative. For this reason, they may be considered a combination of a stop and fricative. Indeed, they are usually written with two symbols: /d/ and /ʒ/ and /t/ and /ʃ/.

Features of Consonants

Using these descriptions of consonants in terms of the manner they are articulated, their maximal constriction (their characteristic place of articulation), and whether or not the vocal folds are vibrating during their production, we can uniquely specify each consonant of English. These descriptive terms are known as *features*. Although the features we have discussed here are articulatory in nature, there are also phonological and phonetic features. We'll return to phonetic features in Chapter 7.

Not only are features useful in describing how different sounds are produced, they also turn out to be useful in characterizing how sounds change in a language over time, how they are acquired by young children, and how they are affected by various speech disorders. Features turn out to be more than mere descriptions of how consonant sounds are articulated; they also have some psychological reality. In other words, at some level, speech sounds or phonemes must also be organized in a similar manner in the human brain. As we'll see, these features are useful for explaining articulation, and they are also relevant for understanding speech perception.

Differences Between Vowel and Consonant Sounds

In some ways, we can think of consonant articulation as more rapid movements superimposed on the slower moving background of vowel production. Of course, such a distinction is not so obvious during ongoing speech production where both sounds are produced very quickly indeed.

A distinction in the type of sound may be a convenient means of organizing the study of speech production, since there is also a difference in perception between consonants and vowels. Many consonants depend on vowels for their production and perception. Vowel sounds can be produced in isolation, but stop consonants require vowels. While we can easily produce an isolated vowel (there are even whole words, such as the article *a* in English, which only consist of a single vowel sound), this is not the case for stop consonants. These consonants are basically impossible to produce without the support of a vowel sound. Even when we say the consonant letters of the alphabet in isolation, we still add a short vowel sound: We write *b, c, d,* but we say /bi/, /si/, /di/. In fact, for even the most purely consonantal sounds we can make, such as when we try just to describe the sound of the letter *k*, we still need at least a little vowel at the end to produce the consonant.

Of course, fricative sounds such as /s/ and /z/ can easily be produced without a vowel, and they can also be sustained for several moments, for as long as we have sufficient breath. Stop consonants cannot be extended in this manner.

The dependence of stop consonants on vowels has a perceptual consequence. In early speech perception experiments, researchers attempted to isolate the individual speech sounds on tape recordings. They found that while they could isolate the vowels, there was essentially no point where they could isolate a single consonant sound. Listeners either heard a whole syllable, including some of the vowel, or they heard some sound which they did not hear as a sound of speech. Researchers had stumbled onto this important perceptual property of speech almost by accident. We will see that this inability to perceptually isolate stop consonants is a property that any adequate theory of speech perception must take into account.

There are several other differences between consonants and vowels that we will briefly consider here. Since stop consonants are dependent on vowels for their production, we can consider vowels in some ways to be more basic speech sounds. In fact, babies usually produce sounds we recognize as vowels earlier than recognizable consonant sounds. This is not to say that babies do not produce any consonant sounds. It means, rather, that there are more recognizable vowel-like sounds than consonant sounds. Interestingly enough, in aphasia—the disorder that can occur after damage to the language areas of the brain—there is evidence that vowel sounds are better preserved, or somewhat less resistant to errors, than are consonant sounds (Ryalls, 1987).

Another difference is that whereas consonant sounds can be produced either with or without the vocal folds vibrating (i.e., voiced consonants like /b/, /d/, /g/ versus unvoiced consonants /p/, /t/, /k/), vowels are almost always produced with the vocal folds vibrating. Vowels require the rapidly vibrating vocal folds for the source of their sound.

Finally, in some ways, vowel preception may be somewhat easier to understand than that for consonants. For this reason we will begin our discussion of speech perception with vowels. You will see that many of the concepts for explaining vowel perception will also be necessary for understanding consonant perception.

We have seen that there are several varieties of consonant sounds in American English. Much of our emphasis in the remainder of this book, however, will be on the stop consonants since it is appropriate for an introduction to the study of speech perception.

In the next chapter, we'll turn our attention away from the way speech sounds are produced to the nature of their sound. In other words, we'll shift the focus from articulation to acoustics. You'll see that having a basic understanding of articulation will help us better comprehend speech acoustics. Speech production provides a framework for understanding acoustic differences between various speech sounds. As in the present chapter, we'll begin with vowels.

Summary

In this chapter you've learned how vowel and consonant sounds are different from each other. The distinguishing articulatory features were presented. They are important since speech perception is organized by the resulting differences in the acoustic signal of speech.

We've learned about the difference between voiced and voiceless sounds and that vowels are more steady-state while consonants are quickly changing. Because of this difference vowels and consonants also require somewhat different perceptual mechanisms.

For Further Reading

Borden, G., Harris, K., & Raphael, L. (1994). *Speech Science Primer: Physiology, Acoustics and Perception of Speech* (3rd Edition). Baltimore, MD: Williams & Wilkins.

Ladefoged, P. (1975). *A Course in Phonetics.* New York: Harcourt Brace Jovanovich.

Singh, S., & Singh, K. (1982). *Phonetics: Principles and Practices* (2nd edition). Austin, TX: Pro-Ed.

REVIEW QUESTIONS

1. Explain the difference between voiced and voiceless sounds.

2. What are the major differences between vowels and consonants?

(continued)

(continued)

3. What is different about fricative sounds compared to stop consonants?

4. Name the features for a /p/ consonant sound.

5. Describe the neutral vowel /ə/ (schwa) in terms of its features.

6. Give the two pieces of evidence that vowel sounds are somehow more basic than stop consonants.

7. Why do you think there are two different types of basic speech sounds? In other words, could a language exist with only consonants or only vowels?

CHAPTER

2

Basic Speech Acoustics

LEARNING OBJECTIVES

In this chapter, you will learn about basic acoustic properties of vowels, about the fundamental frequency of speech,
and how this acoustic event relates to vocal fold vibration.
The basic properties of the source-filter theory of speech
production will be presented, as well as how different positions of the tongue cause the mouth and rest of the vocal
tract to resonate at the different characteristic formant frequencies for each vowel.

This chapter aims to familiarize the reader with harmonics, formant frequencies, and the difference between
the two. It will prepare the reader for an understanding of
the perception of vowels from an acoustic perspective.

Fundamental Frequency

In the last chapter we looked at how speech is produced; in this chapter we will consider the sound qualities of speech. The *acoustics of speech* deals with the study of speech once it is released into the air, not to how it is produced or articulated.

We previously learned that most vowel sounds are voiced, or produced with the vocal folds vibrating in a regular pattern. As vowels are spoken, the regular vibration of the vocal folds also creates a regular pattern in the sound wave. This regular pattern can be seen in Figure 2–1 of a vowel waveform. Our ears react to this pattern generated by the vowel sound and we hear the *pitch* of the vowel. While *fundamental frequency* relates directly to the rate at which the vocal folds vibrate, the term pitch is used when referring to the *perception* of fundamental frequency. As you know, when women or children produce vowel sounds they sound higher in pitch than adult men. The vocal folds of women and children are usually shorter and have less mass than those in adult males, so female vocal folds typically vibrate at a faster rate and produce a higher pitched sound.

The number of times any activity occurs is known as its frequency. Again, when we discuss speech sounds we should remember that the rate at which the vocal folds are vibrating is called the fundamental frequency. The fundamental frequency used to be expressed in cycles per second (cps), which described this frequency in a straightforward manner—one cycle was a complete opening and closing of the vocal folds. Later, this terminology was changed from cps to the modern term *Hertz* in honor of the German physicist Heinrich Hertz (1887–1975).

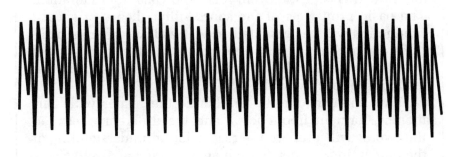

Figure 2–1. Waveform of a vowel sound.

(Hertz are abbreviated Hz. A capital letter is used, because Hertz is a proper name.) For a fundamental frequency of 100 Hz, there are 100 complete openings and closings of the vocal folds in one second.

As mentioned earlier, the rate of vocal fold vibration is continuously varying in ongoing speech (as the vocal folds start up, slow down, and stop activity for the different speech sounds). This rate can be averaged over the length of a spoken sentence. Researchers have found that adult male speakers may have an average fundamental frequency of approximately 100 to 120 Hz. Females typically have a higher average fundamental frequency from about 160 to 200 Hz. Young children may have fundamental frequencies of 300 Hz or even higher.

Recall that the fundamental frequency is the rate at which the vocal folds actually vibrate, while pitch refers to how we hear or perceive the fundamental frequency. This distinction is made between the actual physical vibration of the vocal folds and its perception because there is not an exact correlation between the two. This is especially true for sounds with higher fundamental frequencies. For example, a sound with a fundamental frequency that is twice as high as another sound may not sound twice as high in pitch to our ears.

The fundamental frequency, or rate of vibration of the vocal folds, is one of the sound properties to which our ears react when we hear a vowel. The fundamental frequency is independent of what particular vowel we hear. Different vowels can be produced at the same fundamental frequency, and the same vowel can be spoken at different fundamental frequencies. So fundamental frequency is not the only sound property of vowels, and it is certainly not the one that accounts for the differences in various vowel sounds.

To account for the differences between different vowel sounds it is necessary to recall the source-filter account of speech that was briefly mentioned in Chapter 1. We said that in vowel sounds, at least, the vibrating vocal folds provide the source for these sounds, which is then filtered by the shape of the vocal tract, especially by the position of the tongue. The particular shape of the oral cavity for each of the vowel sounds provides a filter for the sound of the vibrating vocal folds. As this filter is changed, the sound of the vibrating vocal folds is also modified.

The vocal tract is somewhat like a tube which extends from the lips all the way down to the vocal folds. It is not a straight tube, however; there is a sharp bend near the back of the tongue. This bend in the tube allows the tongue to form two small tubes: one in front of the tongue and extending out to the lips, another in back of the tongue and extending down to the vocal folds. Each of the cavities or sections of this tube resonate with the sound of the vibrating vocal folds. There is also a nasal cavity, which may also contribute resonant properties, depending on whether the velopharyngeal port is open or closed. The velum or velopharyngeal port controls whether or not the sound of the vibrating vocal folds enters the nasal cavity.

Of course, this is a simplification of the complex manner in which the acoustic properties of speech are actually generated and modified in the vocal tract. But this simplification allows us to understand the basic principles at play. Readers should remain aware that the actual acoustic results of speech require a more detailed model than is being presented here.

What do we mean by *resonate*? Let's use a simple example. Everyone knows that if we blow air across the top of an empty soft drink bottle, it will make a whistling sound. This is because the air causes the walls of bottle to vibrate or resonate. If we begin to fill the bottle with water, the sound that the bottle now makes sounds higher. This is because the smaller the resonating cavity, the higher the sound that results.

In a very simplified manner, this is similar to what happens in speech. The vibrating vocal folds provide a sound source, which then causes the two cavities, one in front of the tongue, and one behind the tongue, to resonate. These resonances in speech are referred to as *formant frequencies.*

Differences in tongue placement change the formant frequencies and account for the differences between vowels. In order to explain formant frequencies better we need to talk a little more about the fundamental frequency. Even though we said that the vocal folds vibrate at a certain rate, referred to as the fundamental frequency, this is not the only frequency at which energy is present in the sound that results. Owing to the physical properties of vibration, there are also vibrations present at other multiple frequencies of the fundamental. These other multiple frequencies are called *harmonics.* Harmonics are regular multiples of the fundamental frequency. Figure 2–2 gives a representation of a speech

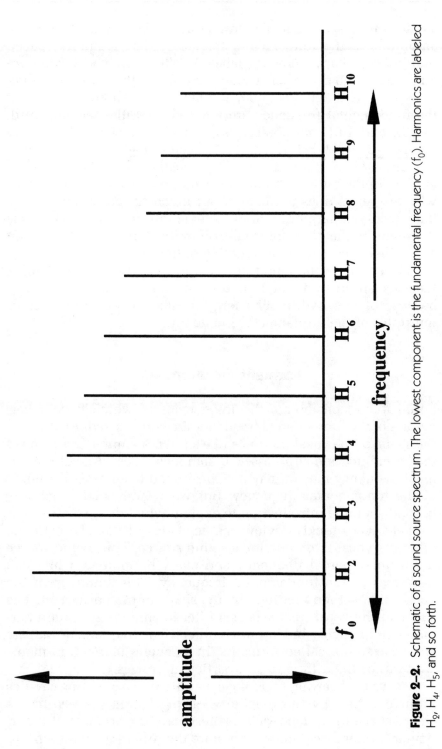

Figure 2–2. Schematic of a sound source spectrum. The lowest component is the fundamental frequency (f_0). Harmonics are labeled H_2, H_3, H_4, H_5, and so forth.

sound source spectrum. The lowest component with the highest amplitude is the fundamental frequency. The regularly spaced multiples or harmonics are labeled. When the vocal folds are vibrating at 100 times per second (100 Hertz), there are also vibrations present at 200, 300, 400, and 500 Hertz. These multiples of the fundamental frequency are referred to as the second, third, fourth, and fifth harmonics, respectively. They are labeled in Figure 2–2 as H2, H3, H4, and H5. Even though there are actually many more harmonics present, typically only harmonics present within the range of human hearing are considered, and this is why the series does not extend out much further. (You can see that the higher harmonics have lower amplitudes. This is because the sound of the vocal folds falls off in intensity at a rate of about 12 decibels per octave, or doubling of frequency.)

The sound of the vibrating vocal folds is thus more complex than its simple rate of vibration, or fundamental frequency, because of this additional energy present at the harmonics or multiples of the fundamental frequency.

Formant Frequencies

Formant frequencies are the frequencies at which certain harmonics of the fundamental frequency are emphasized. As we said, the shape of the vocal tract acts like a filter. It emphasizes some of the harmonics and suppresses or dampens others. Actually, a formant frequency may or may not correspond to an exact harmonic of the fundamental frequency. But we would need to go way beyond a simple introduction to explain why this is so.

Let's just quickly review the acoustics of vowels. First the vibrating vocal folds provide a sound source. This sound source has a fundamental frequency and many harmonics, which are multiples of the fundamental frequency. This sound from the vocal folds is then modified by the shape of the vocal tract. The shape of the vocal tract acts as a filter to emphasize certain harmonic frequencies and suppress others. The frequencies that are emphasized are called formants. In a general manner, formants account for the differences in particular vowels.

As we said earlier, there are generally two resonating cavities formed in part by the tongue when producing vowels. In the simplest manner then, each of these cavities resonate at a particular formant frequency. Therefore the difference between different vowel sounds is accounted for, in the simplest terms, by differences in the first two formant frequencies. Although formant frequencies do not always relate directly to the two cavities formed by the tongue, this is a convenient simplification. For our purposes, we can think of the cavity behind the tongue as accounting for the first formant frequency (abbreviated F_1), while the cavity in front of the tongue accounts for the second formant frequency (abbreviated F_2). Please bear in mind, however, that this is merely a convenient simplification. Formant frequencies in speech do not relate directly to tongue position in such a straightforward manner. But this simplification will serve our purpose to learn the basic relationship between movements of the tongue, mouth, and lips (or *articulation*) and the resulting sound properties.

It is very important not to confuse *harmonics* with *formant frequencies*. Harmonics are multiples of the fundamental frequency. So if we know the fundamental frequency, we also know the harmonics. Such is not the case for the formant frequencies. We need to know the position of the tongue and how it is filtering the sound of the vibrating vocal folds before we can have an idea about the formant frequencies. Remember that varying the fundamental frequency changes the pitch of a vowel, but does not change the vowel we hear (which is dependent on the formant frequencies). We can say the same vowel /i/ (like in *bee*) with a high-pitched voice or with a low voice. It is the formant frequencies that relate to the differences between particular vowel sounds. Formant frequencies result from the position of the tongue or shape of the mouth and they are largely independent of the rate at which the vocal folds are vibrating.

Now for a few more words about vowel articulation and formant frequencies. Everyone who has ever operated a slide whistle realizes that the smaller a cavity, the higher the frequency at which it will resonate. So when the tongue is high and forward in the vocal tract such as for a vowel /i/ (like in the word *see*), we can picture the smaller cavity in the front of the tongue that is responsible for a high second formant frequency (F_2); while the relatively larger cavity posterior to the tongue makes for a low first formant frequency (F_1). In fact, /i/ is the vowel with the highest F_2 and lowest F_1. Consequently, it also has the largest difference between F_1 and F_2.

Moving the tongue lower, the cavity in front of the tongue gets larger and its resonant frequency lowers, while the cavity in back of the tongue gets somewhat smaller so its resonant frequency increases. This general tendency gives us a useful way of remembering the approximate relationship between the first two formants for various vowels.

For the vowel /ɪ/, the tongue is not in quite as high a position as for /i/; therefore the oral cavity is somewhat smaller, and the pharyngeal cavity somewhat larger. Consequently, F_2 is slightly lower, and F_1 slightly higher.

So far, as you have probably noticed, we have only spoken about vowel sounds in this chapter. Formant frequencies are also important for explaining consonant sounds as well. As you'll recall from Chapter 1, the acoustic information that specifies consonants changes much more quickly than for vowels. While vowels are largely determined by relatively stable formant frequencies, many consonant sounds are characterized by the changing portion of formant frequencies. The changing portion of formant frequencies are known as *formant transitions*. They will be discussed in much greater detail in Chapter 4 on the Perception of Consonants.

Summary

The fundamental frequency of a speech sound is the rate at which the vocal folds are set into periodic vibration. We hear this vibration as pitch. This sound is then filtered by the different positions of the vocal tract, which are effected through the various movements of the tongue and lips forming the different vowels. Through resonance, the various articulatory positions result in different characteristic formant frequencies—the first two of which contribute the greatest to speech perception.

In a general manner, a vowel with a high front position of the tongue will result in a vowel with a high F_2 and a low F_1, since the oral cavity in front of the tongue is small and resonates at a high frequency, and the pharyngeal cavity in back of the tongue is relatively large and resonates at a low frequency.

For Further Reading

Kent, R., & Read, C. (1992). *The Acoustic Analysis of Speech.* San Diego, CA: Singular.

Lieberman, P., & Blumstein, S. (1988). *Speech Acoustics, Physiology and Perception*. London: Cambridge University Press.

Speaks, C. (1992). *Introduction to Sound: Acoustics for the Hearing and Speech Sciences*. San Diego, CA: Singular.

REVIEW QUESTIONS

1. Specify the two types of differences between a vowel produced by an adult compared to one made by a child.

2. What is the difference between harmonics and formant frequencies?

3. How does the tongue change in position from a vowel like /i/ to a vowel like /ɪ/?

4. What happens to the first and second formant frequencies with this change from /i/ to /ɪ/?

5. Fundamental frequency can be varied independently of formant frequencies. This is how we can sing the same word or vowel at different notes of the scale. What is another example of how formant and fundamental frequencies are independent from each other?

CHAPTER

3

Perception of Vowels

LEARNING OBJECTIVES

This chapter explains the basic principles involved in the perception of vowels. We'll learn that formant frequecies account for the differences we hear between different vowels and that the ear possesses the ability to isolate these formant frequencies. Since different speakers arrive at different vowel sounds with somewhat different articulatory patterns, it seems that speakers organize speech more along the lines of the acoustic result than they do along the lines of the articulatory patterns that produced this result.

Since women and children have different head sizes and differences in vocal tract length, the vowel sounds they produce are different from those produced by adult male speakers. These differences result in differences in formant frequencies. The other difference between male and female

(continued)

(continued)
speakers (and adults and children) relates to differences in the vocal folds. Since females typically have shorter vocal folds with less mass than males, they also tend to have higher average fundamental frequencies. Children, whose vocal folds are even shorter, usually have even higher fundamental frequencies. We will learn that vowel normalization refers to the perceptual process of factoring out differences due to vocal tract differences.

As stated in Chapter 1, we are going to start with vowels rather than consonants since the perception of vowel sounds is probably somewhat easier to understand. This starting point also makes sense when we consider that consonants are somewhat dependent upon vowels for their perception.

In Chapter 2 it was stated that the position of the tongue changes the shape of the vocal tract which results in different formant frequencies. Formant frequencies account for the differences in the vowels that we hear. But how do we know that it is actually formant frequencies that determine the vowel we hear? It is one thing to say that they result from the position of the tongue and the shape of the vocal tract, but something quite different to state that these frequencies determine what we hear.

One source of evidence about formants comes from machines that can imitate human speech—speech synthesizers. If we sufficiently change the first two formant frequencies of synthesized speech, listeners hear a different vowel sound.

In fact, we have just touched on a very important principle of speech perception in general. Not only do we want to have evidence from production about what contributes to perception, but we also require evidence from perceptual experiments. We know that formant frequencies change when the vowel that is being produced changes. We also know that when we synthesize different formant frequencies, the vowel heard by listeners also changes. It will always be important to have both of these sources of evidence for any conclusions we might draw about speech perception. We want to see evidence both in terms of articulation or production of speech sounds, and from synthesis and listening experiments.

All of this may seem a little abstract at first. We cannot see formants in the air, so how do we know that they are actually there? Well, we can synthesize speech from formant frequencies and show that listeners react to them: When the formants change, so does the sound of the vowel we hear.

Another source of evidence comes from instruments that can make formants visible and measurable. One such device is the *sound spectrograph*. In Figure 3–1 is a spectrogram of the vowel /i/. We can see the first and second formants, which are labeled in the figure. Since this is an introduction to speech perception, spectrograms will not be discussed in much further detail here. You may already be somewhat familiar with spectrograms. In any case, spectrograms are one means of making speech visible and enabling us to measure various acoustic properties of speech such as formant frequencies.

The digital computer, outfitted with specialized programs, is another electronic device used more and more frequently in con-

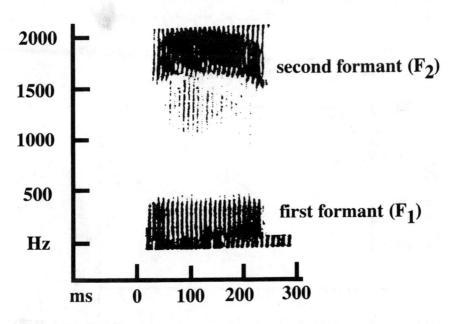

Figure 3–1. Wideband Spectrogram of an /i/ vowel with first and second formant frequency labeled. (Figure adapted from *A Course in Phonetics* by Peter Ladefoged [1975]. Copyright 1975 by Harcourt Brace & Company. Reprinted by permission of the author and publisher.)

temporary speech research. Like a spectrograph, computer-assisted speech analysis may also employ a spectrographic display for analyzing formants, or it may simply produce a spectrum that also indicates formants and other acoustic data of interest. One type of spectrum that is often used in computer-assisted speech analysis is produced by a mathematical procedure (or *algorithm* in computer terminology) called linear predictive coding (LPC). Some LPC displays also list the actual formant frequency values. An example of an LPC display for the vowel /i/ is given in Figure 3–2. As you can see, the formant frequency values are listed along the right side of the printout.

The main advantage of computer-assisted speech analysis over spectrographic analysis is that the computer can usually also be programmed to do a number of other things besides analyze formants. The spectrograph is not adaptable; it is only good for making spectrograms, and it requires that someone interpret the spectrograms and determine the actual formant frequencies. Some computers can even be programmed to synthesize speech as well as measure it. If better programs are developed for analyzing speech, then often even older computers can be outfitted with these newer programs. In

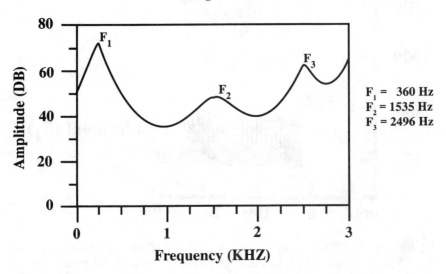

Figure 3–2. LPC (Linear Predictive Coding) spectrum of an /i/ vowel. First (F_1), second (F_2), and third formant (F_3) frequencies listed at right side.

contrast, the analysis routine of the spectrograph cannot be changed—it is hard-wired or permanent. However, the development of digital spectrographs have somewhat blurred the distinction between the spectrograph and the computer.

Basics of Vowel Perception

Now that we know that formant frequencies are present in vowel sounds when they are produced by a speaker, we need to know how listeners extract formants out of the speech that they hear. There is some evidence that the human auditory nerve already reacts directly to formant frequencies (Delgutte, 1980). In most accounts, the ear is probably capable of effecting a kind of basic spectrographic analysis before speech is sent to the brain for further processing.

After sound is captured by our ears it is transformed at the eardrum into mechanical vibrations. These vibrations are transmitted and amplified to some degree by the tiny bones of the middle ear. Then they are transmitted into vibrations of the fluid in the inner ear.

The cochlea—Latinate for shell—resembles the spiral-shaped nautilus shell and is located in the inner ear. We know that, in the fluid-filled cochlea, the nerve cells that react to speech are arranged in order of their frequency sensitivity. This frequency organization is designated *tonotopic* organization.

Without getting into the detailed mechanics of how the ear works, we will simply say that each nerve cell reacts somewhat selectively to the presence of acoustic energy at a certain frequency. So if there is energy present in a formant at a certain frequency, the nerve cell corresponding to that frequency will react and send information about the presence of this energy to the brain. In other words, it seems as if the cochlea functions like a bank of frequency filters.

However, it should be pointed out that there is not much direct evidence of this formant frequency analysis function of the ear. This descriptive model may have to be considerably revised as more direct information about the acoustic analysis performed by the cochlea is obtained.

If the ear can already perform an elementary speech analysis does this mean that we don't need brains to understand speech?

No, of course not. We should qualify that the ear is capable only of a kind of elementary formant frequency analysis. Listeners are very dependent upon how this information is further interpreted by the brain. This point is being brought up here, because it might be easy to overlook the contribution of the brain to speech perception when one considers the marvels of the human ear. Not to detract from the fascinating intricacy of the human ear, but even if the ear were completely capable of perceiving speech by itself, it would still be dependent upon the brain to be capable of reacting to this information. In fact, we will see that the brain still has an awful lot to do with what is actually perceived in speech.

It is the brain that takes the basic acoustic information supplied by the ears and relates it to a specific language. In other words, it is the brain and not the ears that makes speech out of the sounds that we hear. As we will see in later chapters, the brain uses a lot of different kinds of information in interpreting speech sounds.

For example, there is ample evidence that whether a particular sound sequence exists as a word or not in a language has a lot of influence on just what listeners perceive. Listeners may even fill in missing sounds in order to complete a word! But we are getting a bit ahead of ourselves here.

Let us just review what we have learned about the perception of vowels. Vowel sounds are specified by their *formant frequencies*. These formant frequencies relate most directly to the position of the tongue and the length and size of the vocal tract. As we discussed in Chapter 1, vowels are often specified in terms of their characteristic tongue position. A "high front" vowel such as /i/ (in the word *see*), is produced with the tongue tip pointed high toward the hard palate, making a cavity in the front of the vocal tract near the lips and teeth. However, tongue position is not the only factor involved in producing a particular vowel sound. For example, lip rounding has much the same acoustic consequence of making the cavity in front of the tongue larger, as does moving the tongue backward.

There is, in fact, evidence that speakers can arrive at the same acoustic goal using quite different articulations (Ladefoged et al., 1972). For this reason, some researchers have argued that speakers have in mind a particular acoustic goal, and not a particular articulatory configuration, when they are organizing articulation for producing speech. If this is true, it may also in turn imply that listeners monitor the sound of their own speech as a kind of feedback system that tells them about the accuracy of their speech production. This is not to deny that speakers also use sensory information from their articulators in monitoring their speech production.

In any case, once formant frequencies are produced by a speaker they arrive via the air to a listener's ears. In the ear particular nerve cells that are sensitive to certain frequencies react and deliver information about their presence to the brain. We have also described how the sound of the vibrating vocal folds is changed into a particular vowel by the shape of the vocal tract formed by the tongue and, again, how this sound is reacted to by the ears of the listener. What the brain does with this basic sound information will be discussed later.

Vowel Normalization

Having presented a simplified account of how vowels are perceived, we now have to consider a perceptual phenomenon that complicates the picture considerably. If all speakers were about the same size, then once the ear performed its formant analysis the brain could then relate formant frequency values to a particular vowel. In other words, the brain could consult a kind of table of formant frequency values to find which particular vowel is determined by the formant frequencies under consideration.

But the fact is that speakers are very different from each other. Not only are males and females different in the size and mass of their vocal folds, but the length of their vocal tracts can also vary considerably. Even more different from the typical adult male vocal tracts are the vocal tracts of young children. These physical differences in speakers result in considerable differences in the formant frequencies for a particular vowel. Since the resonating cavities that produce formants are smaller for a child, children's formants are also higher in frequency. In other words, the formant frequencies of an /i/ produced by a young child are very different from the formant frequencies for an /i/ produced by an adult male.

In fact there is a considerable degree of overlap of vowel spaces between adults and children. A particular vowel for a child may actually overlap with the formant frequencies that would produce a quite different vowel for an adult. Figure 3–3 illustrates this point. Vowels, plotted by their first and second formant frequencies, for adult males are compared to those for adult females and children.

It is because of this problem in *vowel normalization* that computer systems were developed to recognize speech break down. Yet, research with very young children has provided evidence that they are capable of normalizing vowels for different speakers (Kuhl, 1987; Lieberman, 1984). Infant children can recognize the same vowel across different speakers—despite the acoustic

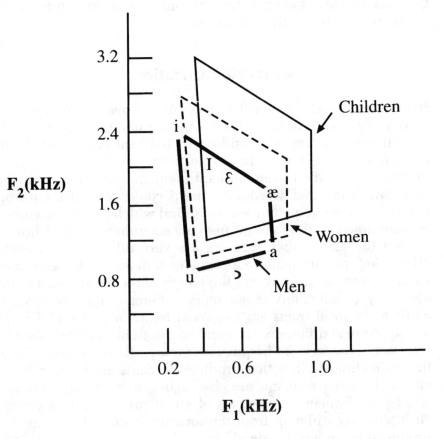

Figure 3–3. Vowel normalization. Representation of differences in vowels according to vocal tract size. (Figure reprinted with permission from Kent & Read (1992), *The Acoustic Analysis of Speech*. San Diego: Singular Publishing Group.

differences. This capacity is present at such a young age in children that researchers have suggested that vowel normalization is innate and present at birth. Sophisticated computer systems are usually not able to perform this same task that infants seem to perform effortlessly.

You might play devil's advocate here and suggest that perhaps we can use visual information about the physical size of a speaker to offset the problem of vowel normalization. In other words, listeners might be able to scale their hypothetical formant frequency tables according to how large or small a speaker looks. This would have to be a fairly complex and instantaneous process, but perhaps it is reasonable to suggest that visual information helps us solve the problem of normalization. But we are also able to understand the speech of people we have never seen before, for example, on tape recordings or over the telephone. In these fairly common situations, we often never see the person to whom we are listening.

Several different proposals attempt to account for how listeners normalize vowels (Neary, 1978; Verbrugge, Strange, Shankweiler, & Erdman, 1976). It is important to recognize that vowel normalization is a necessary component of speech perception and that it is very unlikely that listeners can perform this task on the basis of visual information alone.

It was suggested above that this process may be part of our innate genetic endowment. More will be discussed about the innate capacities that are brought to the task of speech perception later when speech perception in infants is covered in Chapter 11.

Summary

Evidence about the acoustic characteristics of speech come not only from analyzing speech into its basic sound properties, but also from synthesizing speech using its basic acoustic properties as input. Both sources of evidence reveal that the first two formant frequencies determine the various vowel sounds. The ear reacts directly to these formant frequencies, but we still need brains to perceive speech.

Since not all speakers conform to expected patterns of tongue height, some have argued that speech is organized in terms of the acoustic end rather than the articulatory patterns that produce this result.

Because of the significant differences in vocal tracts when comparing adults and children, or even adult males and adult females, vowel normalization is required to account for how the listener ignores these differences that are irrelevant for the same perceived vowel. Since children are capable of vowel normalization at such a young age, many researchers have argued that this capacity is innate.

For Further Reading

Borden, G., Harris, K., & Raphael, L. (1994). *Speech Science Primer: Physiology, Acoustics and Perception of Speech* (3rd edition). Baltimore, MD: Williams & Wilkins.

Lieberman, P., & Blumstein, S. (1988). *Speech Acoustics, Physiology and Perception*. London: Cambridge University Press.

Pisoni, D. (1978). Speech perception. In W. Estes (Ed.), *Handbook of Learning and Cognitive Processes* (Vol. 6.). Hillsdale, NJ: Erlbaum.

REVIEW QUESTIONS

1. Describe the two sources of evidence that formant frequencies are the acoustic property that account for the perception of vowels.

2. Why wasn't the brain considered immediately when vowel perception was described?

3. Why do some researchers think that speech production is planned using acoustic targets rather than an articulatory targets?

4. What is vowel normalization and why do vowels from different speakers need to be normalized?

5. Why does vowel normalization seem to be innate?

CHAPTER

4

Perception of Consonants

LEARNING OBJECTIVES

This chapter aims to make the reader aware that while vowels are dependent on relatively longer duration steady-state portions of formants, much of stop consonant perception depends on the rapidly changing formant transitions. Because these formant transitions for different stop consonants vary greatly according to the vowel sound that follows, there is nothing obvious in the visual representation of speech that can be used to explain the constant perception of a particular consonant sound. This problem is known as the lack of acoustic invariance.

The rest of the chapter attempts to familiarize the reader with various attempts to overcome this problem of acoustic invariance. Locus theory posits that while formant transitions themselves vary greatly across different vowel contexts, these transitions point toward a similar frequency.

As mentioned in Chapter 2, consonant perception is somewhat more complex than vowel perception. Part of this greater complexity stems from the fact that many consonants depend on vowels for their perception. Recall that stop consonant sounds cannot be isolated from vowels without destroying their perception. Figure 4–1 illustrates a formant with the steady-state vowel portion and the consonant *transition* portion labeled. If we look at a two-formant spectrographic representation for a consonant-vowel (CV) syllable such as in Figure 4–2, in this case /di/, we can easily identify the vowel portion. The vowel portion has steady-state or relatively stable formant frequencies. While it is true that the transition is the portion of the acoustic signal that delivers the perception of a consonant, if the audio signal associated with this portion is delivered to listeners they do not hear an isolated consonant. For this portion of the acoustic signal, listeners usually hear a consonant and a short vowel sound. But if we cut back the signal further and further to the left to try and get rid of the vowel sound, eventually the sound of the consonant disappears. The sound that remains no longer sounds like speech, but rather like some chirplike noise.

Let us take a look at the transition portion of these spectrographic representations. We see that the formant transitions change quickly and then smooth out and become stable. These formant "tails" are known as *formant transitions*. In contrast with the steady-state portion of the formant, formant transitions change very quickly in frequency. Even though we cannot isolate the consonant, the acoustic correlates of the consonant are still

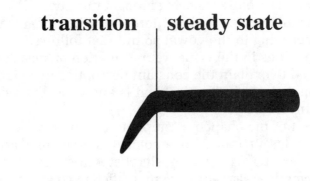

Figure 4–1. Schematic of a transition and steady-state portion of a formant frequency transition.

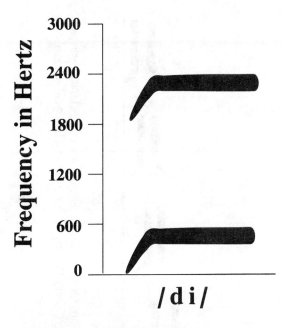

Figure 4–2. Schematic of first two formant frequency pattern for a /di/ syllable. (Adapted with permission from Liberman, Cooper, Shankweiler, & Studdert-Kennedy [1967]. Copyright 1967 by the American Psychological Association.)

somehow present in this portion of the signal. In fact, it is often taught that consonant perception is delivered by these rapidly changing formant transitions.

However, to understand consonant perception we need to look at the same consonant produced with different vowels, as in Figure 4–3. If we hypothesize that consonant perception is dependent on the formant transition portion of the spectrogram, we see that this portion changes considerably when the same consonant is produced with different vowels. In fact, there is nothing constant between the formant transitions from the production of /d/ in front of one vowel and /d/ in front of another vowel. Yet, listeners still have a constant perception of /d/ even though the different vowel sounds change the transition portions of the signal dramatically. In other words, the formant transition patterns look very different when the /d/ consonant occurs in front of various vowels.

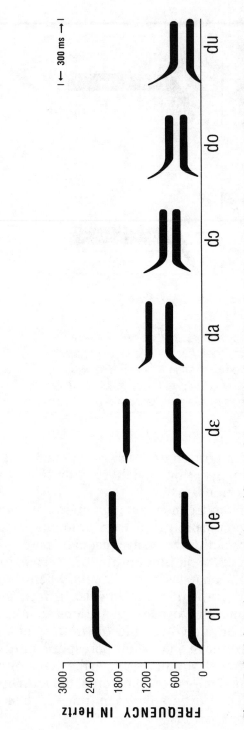
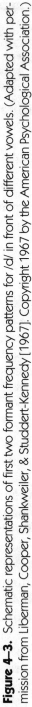

Figure 4-3. Schematic representations of first two formant frequency patterns for /d/ in front of different vowels. (Adapted with permission from Liberman, Cooper, Shankweiler, & Studdert-Kennedy [1967]. Copyright 1967 by the American Psychological Association.)

40

This problem of the lack of something constant in the spectrographic representation that could signal the consonant is known as the lack of *acoustic invariance*. There is nothing acoustically invariant or constant between this consonant produced in different vowel contexts. We are now going to spend some time discussing various proposals that have been offered for solving this important problem in speech perception. Before we do so, take a few minutes to understand this problem. Look at how different the same consonant pattern is in front of different vowels. If these formant patterns are an accurate representation of the acoustic information used for speech perception, then what portion of the consonant portion of pattern remains constant in front of the various vowels?

One of the first proposals that was offered to solve this problem was called *locus theory*. Basically this theory offered an ingenious solution. Even though there was nothing constant in the formant transition patterns themselves between the same consonant produced in different vowel contexts, the second formant frequency transitions all seem to be pointing toward the same frequency. That is, if we were to extend the formant transitions back in time, there would be a point to the left where they would eventually cross each other. This locus point, or frequency towards which the formant transitions are aimed, is known as the *locus*. It is approximately 1800 Hertz in Figure 4–3. Since this point seems to be the same across different vowels, it may be the solution for the problem of invariance. Eureka!

But if we stop and think a little more carefully about this proposed solution, we will quickly discover a considerable drawback. Basically what we would be stating with locus theory is that consonant perception is based on a frequency *which is never actually present in the signal*. This is, at best, a very abstract theory. At worst, it is a little like hocus-pocus. The actual situation is even worse because speech synthesis experiments have revealed that if this locus frequency is actually included in the acoustic signal, perception is altered—it is no longer a good /d/ sound. Also the frequency toward which the formant transitions point, turns out not to be exactly the same from vowel to vowel.

We have just covered in a simplified form the basic problem outlined in a classic article on speech perception entitled "Perception of the Speech Code" (Liberman, Cooper, Shankweiler, & Studdert-Kennedy, 1967). Essentially at this point in the search, its authors give up looking for invariance in the acoustic signal. While they point out that it might still be contained within the acoustic signal, since they have not been able to find it there, they look elsewhere. The solution that they favor is in articulation. These researchers argue that since the motor commands that are sent to the articulators to produce a /d/ must be the same even in different vowel contexts, these motor commands might be used for speech perception. This theory, called the *motor theory of speech perception*, will be considered in more detail in Chapter 6.

Without offering more of a solution to the problem of invariance at this point, we shall now turn our attention to some other important attributes of speech that are necessary to comprehend in order to better explain its perception. We hope you will still remain curious about solving the problem of invariance, since we have not yet discussed every possible solution.

Early on, speech researchers thought of speech units as "beads on a string." That is, they thought that it would be possible to isolate the individual units of speech, like pearls on a necklace. They thought that even though speech looked like one continuous entity, if they were somehow able to cut the string, the individual units, the consonants and vowels, would become apparent. As we discussed, speech researchers were able to isolate vowels, but they were not successful in isolating stop consonants. Because of this, they began to think of speech as *encoded*. That is, they began to think of vowels and consonants as being squeezed together, perhaps in syllable-sized units.

Perhaps a word about the way we write words is in order here. Most likely, one of the main reasons that early researchers thought that *phonemes*, or speech units perceived as a single distinctive unit, could be isolated from each other is because when we write words, there are individual discrete units or letters of the alphabet that are used to spell the whole word. Even when we join letters together, such as in cursive writing, we can still visually isolate what strokes form which particular letters. In the alphabet, vowel letters are just as independent as are consonant letters. So the writing version, the spelling or *orthography* of a word, gives the impression that consonants and vowels can be isolated into discrete individual units. However, the difference between consonants and vowels is perhaps the most fundamental aspect of the manner in which speech differs from writing. Yet, it is logical to think that speech and writing are similar because we can pronounce words from their written versions.

It is important to point out another important difference between writing and speech. We all know that there is a definite limit to how fast we can read and write. While there are a great deal of individual differences, there is still an upper limit to how fast people can write and read. Of course, some highly skilled people can type words at a rate considerably faster than they can write. And this rate can sometimes be rather impressive. Yet even the fastest typists cannot type at anything approaching the rate at which most speakers can produce speech. Usually we can also understand speech just as fast as it can be produced. Certainly you have had the experience of listening to speech that has been "compressed" or accelerated—for example, playing a tape or a record at a faster speed than which it was recorded. It is rather remarkable that, even though the voice gets higher, we can often still understand what is being said even though it is played much faster than when originally spoken.

In fact the rate at which individual units can be presented in speech is phenomenal. Speech can be understood at rates of about 30 phonemes per second (Liberman et al., 1967). What is remarkable about this rate of presentation is that if some other series of individual sounds were being presented at so fast a rate, they would merge together into a single undistinguishable sound. We can consider the moving pictures for an analogous effect. We know that a film is actually made up of static pictures. Yet when they are presented one after another at a certain rate of speed, the static images become continuous and we no longer see the individual static images. The rate at which the individual pictures become continuous is called the *critical flicker*.

In the auditory realm, when sounds like different bells are presented at too fast a rate, they also become indistinguishable and we hear a continuous buzz rather than individual discrete sounds. What is amazing about speech, is that it can be presented at rates that would become a buzz if it were composed of some other sounds. For this reason, speech is considered to be a special type of sound. As we pointed out above, researchers have described speech as encoded. That is, the individual units or phonemes of speech are squeezed together or blended such that one portion of the signal may actually be delivering information about more than one unit at a time. This encoding in speech perception is similar to the concept of coarticulation in the production of speech. *Coarticulation* in speech production refers to the fact that the articulation for one phoneme impinges on the articulation of another. In other words the articulators are usually already beginning to move toward the position necessary for the next phoneme, even before they have completed their movement for the present phoneme.

Finally, we will turn our attention to considering the unit of speech perception. The fact that speech units are squeezed together or encoded has led some researchers to consider that perception may depend on units other than phonemes such as syllables. It may indeed turn out that speech perception takes place in syllable-sized units rather than phoneme-sized units. Although syllable-sized units are useful for dealing with the encoded nature of speech, they do not solve the problem of invariance that was presented earlier. We will not consider anything further about the size of the units of speech perception. But you should be aware that this is still an unresolved issue in research on speech perception.

There are many more proposals for how speech perception takes place than will be discussed in this book. There are Autonomous Search Models, Fuzzy Logic Models, and the Interactive Activation Model, to name a few. All of the models possess various characteristics such as whether they are active or passive search models, whether the search is autonomous or interactive, and whether the search proceeds from sound to meaning (bottom-up) or whether meaning also has an influence in the search (top-down). Rather than give an exhaustive treatment of speech perception theory, we have chosen to present two influential models in their approximate chronological order of development. In this manner, the reader will have the basic information about speech perception necessary to comprehend these other recent models as well as a rough idea of the history of the endeavor to understand speech perception. Since models of speech perception are presently in a state of constant flux, it would be impossible to provide an accurate and exhaustive account. We have opted to provide the reader with the basic information, which the reader can supplement with more detailed information from research journals where speech perception models are actively debated.

In conclusion, we have touched on two important aspects of speech in this chapter. First of all we have discussed the problem of invariance. Because of the problem of invariance we cannot extend the rather simple spectrographic representation used to explain vowel perception to the perception of consonants. We will consider another proposal to solve this problem of invariance in the next chapter. Next we considered some of the special aspects of speech—the fact that it can be presented at a faster rate of speed than another sound signal and still retain its perceptual integrity. Finally we discussed the encoded nature of speech units both in their production and consequently for their perception.

Summary

Whereas it is the steady-state portions of formants that determine vowels, it is the rapidly changing formant transitions that help specify consonant sounds. When consonant sounds are considered with the vowels which must follow them, there is nothing obvious that is constant or invariant that could be used to explain perception of the same consonant. Although these formant transitions point to a similar starting frequency or locus, it does not seem logical to explain speech perception in terms of a frequency that is not actually present in the acoustic signal. The encoded nature of speech is considered. Speech is very different from written language, in which individual letters can easily be isolated. Whereas vowel sounds can be isolated, stop consonant sounds cannot.

For Further Reading

Borden, G., Harris, K., & Raphael, L. (1994). *Speech Science Primer: Physiology, Acoustic and Perception of Speech* (3rd edition). Baltimore, MD: Williams & Wilkins.

Liberman, A., Cooper, F., Shankweiler, D., & Studdert-Kennedy, M. (1967). Perception of the speech code. *Psychological Review, 74*, 431–461.

Pisoni, D. (1978). Speech perception. In W. Estes (Ed.), *Handbook of Learning and Cognitive Processes* (Vol. 6). Hillsdale, NJ: Erlbaum.

REVIEW QUESTIONS

1. What happens when we try to isolate stop consonant sounds from an audio recording of speech?

2. What are some of the important differences between the written and spoken forms of language that were discussed in this chapter?

3. Briefly explain the problem of acoustic invariance.

4. What is the problem with locus theory as a solution for the problem of acoustic invariance?

CHAPTER

5

Categorical Perception

LEARNING OBJECTIVES

The goal of this chapter is to acquaint the reader with categorical perception—one of the important ways in which the
perception of speech is different from the perception of
other sounds such as musical tones. Voice onset time (VOT)
is the parameter used to illustrate categorical perception.
Some of the attributes of categorical perception are discussed, as well as some of the reasons why it facilitates
ongoing speech perception.

Voice Onset Time Production

In this chapter we are going to consider another difference
between the perception of vowels and consonants. This difference is *categorical perception*. In order to do so, we are going to
concentrate the discussion on voiced versus voiceless—a sound

contrast in consonants. *Voicing*, or absence of voicing, pertains to whether or not the vocal folds are vibrating. In general terms, in a voiced fricative like /z/ the vocal folds are vibrating, whereas in its voiceless counterpart /s/, they are not. You can actually feel this difference if you sustain a /z/ (ZZZZZZZ) and put your finger against the place in your throat where your vocal folds are located (in males the so-called Adam's apple, which is not so prominent on the throat of females). You can feel a vibration from the outside due to the vibration of the vocal folds inside. In /s/ (SSSSSSS) you do not feel this vibration. Note that the presence or absence of vocal fold vibration, or voicing, is the only difference between the way we produce each of these two phonemes.

Many word pairs in English are differentiated only by the presence or absence of voicing in their initial consonants. Examples include *big* and *pig*, *dot* and *tot*, and *coo* and *goo*. There are also pairs that are only different by the absence or presence of voicing in the final consonant, such as *mob* and *mop*, and *kid* and *kit*.

While it is mostly true that the presence or absence of voicing is what differentiates stop consonants like /b/ and /p/, stop consonants are somewhat different from the fricatives /z/ and /s/. That is, stop consonants depend on a vowel for their production, as was pointed out in Chapters 1 and 4. Since all vowels are voiced, sooner or later the vocal folds are set into vibration, even for so-called voiceless stop consonants like /p/, /t/, and /k/. Actually then, the difference between voiced and voiceless stop consonants is not absolute but rather is one of timing. In voiced stop consonants the voicing begins much earlier, almost at the same moment that they are released from the lips. In other words, the voicing begins almost simultaneously when the occlusion of the airstream is released.

In contrast, there is a delay in the onset of vocal fold vibration after the occlusion is released in the case of voiceless consonants. So you see that the difference between voiced and voiceless stop consonants is actually one of the relative timing of the onset of vocal fold vibration. This timing difference is referred to as the *voice onset time*, which is abbreviated VOT. Lisker and Abramson (1964) were the first researchers to define VOT and to investigate how it is produced in a variety of languages.

Voiced stop consonants have a relatively short VOT (in Lisker & Abramson's terminology a short *voice lag*,) whereas voiceless consonants have a longer VOT (long voice lag). In many languages, the vibration of the vocal folds for voiced consonants may actually begin *before* the consonant is released. In this case, we speak of negative VOT (i.e., *prevoicing*, or what Lisker & Abramson called *voice lead*).

Conveniently enough, there is an acoustic marker for the release of the consonant. When the obstruction in the vocal tract is removed and the mouth is opened, there is a sudden release of acoustic energy called the burst or transient. When it is isolated from the surrounding sounds, this burst can be heard as a tapping or popping sound. It can usually be seen on a spectrogram as a very short interval of high-frequency energy. It generally looks like a sudden burst of high-frequency energy—hence its name. Since the vocal folds are not yet in motion at the release, the acoustic energy of a burst is not regular or periodic, but is seen as noise spread through a wide range of frequencies.

These days, VOT is measured more often on a computer-assisted oscillographic display as in Figure 5–1, rather than from a spectrogram. This is because we can place markers or cursors at the point associated with the release and listen to the burst to make sure that we are at the right point. Then we can place another cursor at the onset of vocal fold vibration, and the computer will automatically display this difference in time. The advantage of the computer system over the spectrograph is that we can listen to the burst to make sure it is where we think it is, from visual inspection of the waveform. Once the VOT interval is isolated visually by the placement of cursors, the VOT value

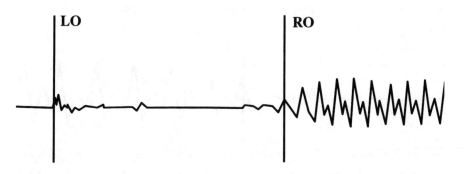

Figure 5–1. VOT measure for a /p/. The left cursor is placed at burst, and the right cursor is placed at the highest point of the first cycle of vocal fold vibration.

is displayed in milliseconds. On the spectrogram we can no longer hear the acoustic signal once it has been removed from the spectrograph, and we have to interpolate the VOT. Since this time interval is quite short it is easy to make a large mistake in measuring the voice onset time on a spectrogram. Most computer-based speech analysis programs allow the user to enlarge the relevant portion of the acoustic signal, and in this manner a somewhat more accurate measure of the VOT is probably obtained.

In Figure 5–1 a VOT measure for a /p/ is illustrated. At the left cursor, you can see the burst associated with the release of the consonant, and at the right cursor you can see the onset of vocal fold vibration. Figure 5–2 illustrates the VOT for a /b/, and you can see that the measure for this voiced consonant is much shorter than for the voiceless /p/. That is, the distance between the arrows in the figures is shorter for /b/ than for /p/.

Figure 5–3 represents VOT productions for a single speaker of American English for repeated productions of different words beginning with either a /t/ or a /d/. You can see that there are essentially two distinct areas or *VOT categories*, one for /t/ and one for /d/, even though there is also a considerable amount of variation. In other words, the VOT productions are fairly spread out over a range of values. In fact, the productions with the longest VOT in this figure is about +95 ms, while the shortest VOT is about − 75 ms. In this case then, there is a difference of 170 ms between the longest and shortest VOT production. However, most of the voiced productions (here, the d's) cluster between 0 and 25 ms, while the voiceless productions (the t's)

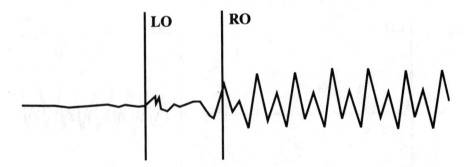

Figure 5–2. VOT measure for a /b/. The left cursor is placed at burst, and the right cursor is placed at the highest point of the first cycle of periodic vocal fold vibration.

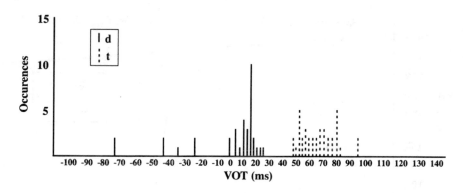

Figure 5–3. VOT productions of a single normal adult speaker of American English for words beginning with /d/ and /t/. (Figure adapted with permission from Blumstein, Cooper, Goodglass, Statlender, & Gottlieb, [1980]. Production Deficits in Aphasia: A Voice Onset-Time Analysis. *Brain and Language, 9,* 153–170. Copyright 1980 by Academic Press.)

cluster between 50 and 80 ms. Although negative VOT productions are not typical of most English productions, almost every voiced stop production typically has a negative VOT in a language like French and many other languages including Spanish, Dutch, and German (Lisker & Abramson, 1967).

Notice that in these productions, the speaker produced two discrete categories with no overlap. It is as if the speaker avoids productions between 30 and 50 ms, since such productions could be perceptually ambiguous between /t/ and /d/.

Voice Onset Time Perception

Now let us consider VOT perception. In Figure 5–4 we have perception results for one listener on a VOT continuum. In this continuum, the VOT has been manipulated from −73 ms to +77 ms. The line at the top left of the diagram represents what percentage of the time the stimuli with that particular VOT value was heard as a /d/, while the line for /t/ is at the top right. You can see that all the VOTs from −73 ms to 0 ms were heard as "d." The stimuli at +11 ms was heard 90% of the time as /d/. We can see that the perception is already beginning to change. As soon as the VOT production changes to +22 ms, suddenly the perception changed completely to 100% /t/. What is important to con-

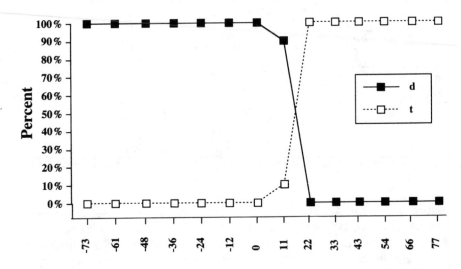

Figure 5–4. Identification functions of a single listener for VOT continuum from /d/ to /t/ in approximately 11 ms steps. Each stimulus is presented 10 times each in random order.

sider is that all of the VOTs from −73 ms to 0 ms were heard as /d/, while a small change of 0 from +22 ms changed the perception from a /d/ to a /t/. In fact listeners do not really hear much of a difference between these stimuli within the /d/ category. There is actually much more physical difference in VOT between the first stimuli of −73 ms and the last 100% /d/ stimuli at 0 ms (i.e., 73 ms), than there is between 0 ms and 22 ms where the perception changes completely (i.e., 22 ms). This example demonstrates that perception does not always adhere to the physical scale. This insensitivity to differences within a category, but keen sensitivity to cross-category differences, is referred to as *categorical perception*.

Categorical Perception

Usually listeners can *discriminate* many more different sounds than they can absolutely *identify*. For example in music we can hear the differences between many finer distinctions in pitch than we can identify with a particular note. Liberman and colleagues (1967) have estimated that we can discriminate about 1200 different pitches, but we can only absolutely identify about 7! This huge discrepancy between discrimination and identification is typical of the perception for most sounds. But for certain sound differences relevant to speech, like that of the VOT dimension (for which perception is categorical), listeners can only discriminate accurately about as many sounds as they can identify. In other words, listeners are not able to put a label on differences in VOT within a category, and they don't even discriminate these differences in a reliable manner. This insensitivity to within-category differences is made formal in the way that we put a single label (such as "d") on all the sounds within a particular VOT category.

Although we have spoken only about the VOT dimension here in our discussion of categorical perception, there is also categorical perception for the differences that lead to a change in place-of-articulation (e.g., the difference between /b/, /d/, and /g/). Here again, listeners do not hear a sound that becomes gradually less and less /b/-like and then becomes more and more /d/-like. Rather they hear pretty much similar /b/'s until all of a sudden their perception changes abruptly to /d/.

Yet, if vowels are synthesized with similar small steps of change in formant frequencies between them, listeners are aware of these small changes. They generally hear even rather small differences in the formants that make up vowels, and the perception does not change in an abrupt manner as we saw for consonants. As the formant frequencies that specify vowels gradually change, the perceptual quality of the vowels also gradually change. In general, the perception for vowels is gradual or continuous, and not categorical. This is another manner in which vowels and consonants differ.

While generally vowel stimuli do not produce the categorical perception effects seen with stop consonant stimuli, there are special conditions under which vowels seem to be perceived in a more categorical manner. If vowels are edited down to a very brief duration, if they are masked with noise so that they are difficult to perceive, or if the amount of difference between vowel stimuli is reduced, then the categorical effect increases.

In Chapter 11 on infant perception, we will show that categorical perception seems to be present from birth in humans. Categorical perception is another manner in which speech is thought to be special. Listeners are generally aware of fairly small changes in nonspeech sounds such as musical notes. The advantage that categorical perception confers to speech is to allow listeners to hear in terms of the phonemes of their particular language and to ignore nonessential variation within a category (Werker, 1989).

There has been quite a bit of controversy surrounding the concept of categorical perception and whether it is exclusively a property of speech. Categorical perception has been demonstrated for certain nonspeech sounds (Cutting, 1972). But it is not crucial for our purposes here whether or not it can be demonstrated for nonspeech sounds. Categorical perception is characteristic of certain speech sound distinctions, and it is generally not found for most nonspeech sounds. It is thought to represent one of the ways in which the human perceptual system has become specially adapted for the perception of speech. It represents one means of coping with the enormous amount of variation between different productions of the same sound typically found in human speech. It gives us one means of coping with this variation in real time—irrelevant differences between different productions of the same speech sound are ignored in order to speed up the recognition process. Otherwise, we might take a lot of time deciding about which phoneme to assign to certain sounds if they sounded ambiguous. Categorical perception circumvents a lot of such potential guess work, since we usually do not even hear speech sounds to be ambiguous. It represents one of the perceptual mechanisms humans have apparently developed for coping with the tremendous amount of information presented at the very rapid rate of transmission typically found for human speech.

Summary

Categorical perception represents one of the essential differences between the perception of speech and other sounds. It is one of the ways in which perception seems to have been specially adapted for speech. While listeners can usually discriminate many more sound differences than they can reliably identify, in categorical perception listeners can only accurately discriminate about as many differences in speech sounds as they can identify. Presumably, this allows listeners to perceive speech at a much more rapid rate than other sound sequences.

For Further Reading

Liberman, A., Cooper, F., Shankweiler, D., & Studdert-Kennedy, M. (1967). Perception of the speech code. *Psychological Review, 74*, 431–461.

Lieberman, P., & Blumstein, S. (1988). *Speech Acoustics, Physiology and Perception*. London: Cambridge University Press.

Pisoni, D. (1978). Speech perception. In W. Estes (Ed.), *Handbook of Learning and Cognitive Processes* (Vol. 6). Hillsdale, NJ: Erlbaum.

REVIEW QUESTIONS

1. Explain the difference between a voiced stop consonant like /b/ and its voiceless counterpart /p/ in terms of voice onset time.

2. What are the special characteristics of categorical perception? How is it different from the perception of non-speech sounds?

3. Are vowels perceived categorically?

4. Can listeners be led to perceive vowels categorically? How?

5. What is the purpose of categorical perception?

CHAPTER

6

Motor Theory of Speech Perception

LEARNING OBJECTIVES

The goal of this chapter is to explain the basic concepts behind the motor theory of speech perception which dominated the field for many years, to discuss its strengths and weaknesses, and to present evidence for and against it. The reader should gain a basic understanding of motor theory and be better prepared to grasp current research in this area. The somewhat related theory of analysis-by-synthesis is presented and compared to motor theory. The concept of template matching is also introduced.

In reading this chapter, the reader should also gain a better understanding of just what phenomena must be accounted for in a comprehensive theory of speech perception.

Motor Commands as a Solution
to Acoustic Invariance

You will recall from Chapter 4 the problem of acoustic invariance—that is, when a stop consonant is produced in various vowel contexts there is no apparent consistent acoustic cue that can account for its constant perception. After consideration of various means to resolve this problem (notably the locus theory, see Chapter 4), the researchers who originally pointed out this problem essentially gave up their search for answers in the acoustic signal itself.

Instead they proposed that, since there must be invariant or constant motor commands to the articulators to produce the same consonant in different vowel contexts, the perceptual process could exploit these motor commands. Motor commands are the neural messages that the brain sends to set the articulators in motion to produce speech. Hence the term *motor* theory of speech perception. Although there are several different versions of motor theory, here we will consider the one most commonly referred to by this term. As the researchers who proposed this theory stated in their original paper: "Though we cannot exclude the possibility that a purely auditory decoder exists, we find it more plausible to assume that speech is perceived by processes that are also involved in its production" (Liberman, Cooper, Shankweiler, & Studdert-Kennedy, 1967, p. 452).

Motor theory does capture the insight of the important link between speech production and speech perception pointed out in Chapter 1. But it is one thing to posit that speech production offers important cues about speech perception which can be used by listeners, and quite another to state that it forms the basis for speech perception. The former is a "weak" version of motor theory, while the latter is a "strong" version of the theory. While strong parsimonious theories are preferred in the scientific method, there are some serious drawbacks to a strong version of the motor theory, which indicate that a weakened version may be more appropriate. However, it should also be pointed out immediately that motor theory represents an important hypothesis about speech perception that still has many adherents decades after its initial proposal. Even if motor theory were eventually to fall out of favor, no basic introduction to speech perception should forgo its consideration.

If correct, or even partially correct, the motor theory has especially wide implications for speech-language pathology and audiology, and therefore should be carefully considered by students of these fields. This is true even if, at first blush, the idea that speech perception is based on the motor commands that produce speech seems to defy intuitive logic. Two of the original formulators of this theory have since proposed a revised version of the theory (Liberman & Mattingly, 1985), which we will also consider.

Evidence Against Motor Theory

One problem with the theory is that it has never been made explicit just how listeners would "extract" motor commands from the acoustic signal. In other words, it is not at all clear how a person could make the link between acoustic speech signals in the air and the motor commands in a speaker's brain that would have produced such signals.

Perhaps the major drawback to the theory is that, once the problem of how listeners perform the link between the acoustic signal and the motor commands is solved, why would listeners not simply go directly to phonemes? In other words, it does not seem any more complicated to go from the acoustic signal directly to phonemes, than it does to go from the acoustic signal to motor commands and then to phonemes. It is not clear why perception would still have to be mediated by motor commands, once the theory has the power to "decode" the acoustic signal. The link from acoustic signal to phoneme seems somewhat more direct than an intervening link between the acoustic signal and motor commands to the speech articulators.

Thus, in a certain sense, motor theory displaces the problem. We are still left with the problem of explaining how the relevant information is deduced from the acoustic signal. In the case of the motor theory, listeners are presumably extracting motor commands. But just how these motor commands are linked up with the acoustic signal remains an important problem, presuming that listeners are not capable of having access to motor commands from a speaker other than via the acoustic signal. (To take the point to an extreme—as listeners we don't have modems that physically link us up with the motor commands in a speaker's brain.)

Once the motor theory of speech perception was formulated, researchers began to look for the invariance that was supposed to be present in motor commands. One means of investigating this theory was to look directly at the neural signals to the muscles of articulation via electromyography (EMG). In electromyography, electrodes are either placed on the surface of the skin directly above muscles or, for even more accurate recordings, inserted directly into muscles. These electrodes can then record directly the electrical impulses that trigger muscle contractions.

But in the early studies, EMG traces appeared to be just as variable as the acoustic signal. It is true that EMG techniques were in their infancy and perhaps part of the variability seen was due to irrelevant "noise" that was picked up from other muscle activity. However, early EMG studies certainly did not support a strict interpretation of motor theory.

One piece of evidence that seems to go against motor theory is the fact that patients with Broca's aphasia (damage to the speech center of the brain) who have serious motor problems in producing speech do not seem to have as significant a problem with speech perception. At least their speech perception does not seem to be perturbed to the degree that would be expected from a tight link between production and perception (see Blumstein,1978, for review). Furthermore, patients with Wernicke's aphasia (resulting from a lesion in another portion of the brain) who do not usually experience motor speech problems typically seem to have more difficulties with speech perception than those with Broca's aphasia. However, it should also be pointed out that in several experiments the speech perception abilities of Wernicke's aphasics have not been shown to be statistically inferior to those of Broca's aphasics (Blumstein, Goodglass, & Baker, 1977; Ryalls, 1987).

Evidence for Motor Theory

On the positive side of the motor theory, there continues to remain undeniable evidence that speech perception and speech production are somehow linked. For example, you may have had the experience of watching foreigners move their lips as they attempt to understand the words of an unfamiliar spoken message. It is as if they need to be able to produce the sounds, before they can understand them. Phoneticians often begin with mastery of production of a new phoneme before they attempt to transcribe it in a consistent manner. The fact that some people with profound hearing losses can "read" speech from the lips and face also argues for a link between motor speech gestures and phonemes.

Another piece of evidence that supports the link between speech production and perception that should not be overlooked comes from the so-called *McGurk effect* (named after the person who first observed it). In the McGurk effect, listeners combine visual information on speech production with auditory information. In the researchers' own words: "on being shown a film of a young woman's talking head, in which repeated utterances of the syllable [ba] had been dubbed onto lip movements for [ga], normal adults reported hearing [da]" (McGurk & MacDonald, 1976, p. 746). In other words, listeners make an agglomeration of the auditory and visual modalities and perceive a place-of-articulation that is intermediate between the two delivered by seeing and listening.

Television ads often exploit this very human tendency to correlate a visual and an auditory signal that are timed together. When an animal's lips move in sync with a voice, for example, as listeners we automatically infer a "talking" animal. This principle can even apply to inanimate objects that we know very well cannot actually speak. Motor theory accounts for the way this visual information influences speech perception. Any alternative theory will also have to account for these phenomena, which are naturally accommodated in motor theory. But perhaps a weaker version of motor theory, which still captures the influence of production in perception, is in order. In a weakened version, speech perception would not be driven by (or entirely based on) motor commands.

Revised Motor Theory

The revised version, which two of the original developers of motor theory have set forth, attempts to take into consideration new information gathered since the original theory was first developed (Liberman & Mattingly, 1985). Specifically, there are two new developments that the newer version of the theory seeks to take into account. The first is the concept of *modules* or specialized subprocessing routines in the brain (Fodor, 1983). The idea for the basis of modules is that the brain has developed specialized areas for treating certain perceptual information. These areas act somewhat independently of other brain processing. Although the localization of these hypothetical modules within the brain remains largely unknown, the concept of modules has proven to be a powerful construct for explaining the function of the brain.

The second development that is accounted for in the revised motor theory is the discovery of *duplex perception*. In duplex perception, transitions for F_1 are presented to one ear, while those for F_2 are presented to the other ear. What some listeners hear is both speech and nonspeech at the same time. In other words, in duplex perception the same acoustic information can be simultaneously processed in both a speech and nonspeech mode. The authors of the revised motor theory view the fact that these two modes of processing can exist at the same time as powerful evidence that a specialized perceptual mode for treating speech has evolved in human beings—one that exploits the invariant relationship between motor gestures and the acoustic signal in order to decode speech. As the authors of the revised theory state themselves: "According to the revised theory, phonetic information is perceived in a biologically distinct system, a 'module' specialized to detect the intended gestures of the speaker that are the basis for phonetic categories" (Liberman & Mattingly, 1985, p. 1).

Even after several decades of intensive investigation, a great amount of research is still being devoted to the issue of just how speech perception is accomplished. Although motor theory is one of the more popular contending theories, there is presently no consensus on a single theory of speech perception. For this reason, and the fact that this is a basic introduction, we will consider only a few more theories in this book.

Analysis-by-Synthesis

A theory related to motor theory is that of *analysis-by-synthesis*. In some accounts, analysis-by-synthesis is only a slightly different version of the motor theory. In this theory once again perception is somewhat based on production. Listeners are hypothesized to decode the acoustic signal by internally generating matching signals. The signal that provides the best match is the one "perceived" by the listener. Perhaps the most important difference between analysis-by-synthesis and motor theory is that the former does not stipulate that it is specifically motor commands that mediate perception. These two theories are similar enough to be considered together here. However, analysis-by-synthesis also requires a matching process with the acoustic signal. Even though we will not go into further detail on analysis-by-synthesis, we will consider how this matching process might take place, because it may offer some insight into the speech perception process.

One account for the means by which this matching between acoustic signal and phonemes may occur is actually borrowed from the study of visual perception. The concept of internalized recognition patterns, or *templates*, has proven to be a powerful metaphor for explaining visual perception. We can take common letter stencils for an illustration of how these templates might work. We all know that letter stencils are useful for producing uniform and highly readable letter patterns. But you probably have not thought about using this same stencil for letter recognition as well. Once a letter has been produced, the stencil could also be used to discover which letter it was. Figure 6–1 illustrates this process.

We could go through the stencil, letter by letter, attempting to match up the written letter with the stencil pattern that may have produced it. The best match, or the pattern of holes that is most completely filled in, is provided by the correct letter. You might already realize that this means of discovering which letter was printed is a rather lengthy process. In fact, we cannot be sure that we have the best match until we have gone through the whole alphabet.

A similar drawback was pointed out by the original proponents of analysis-by-synthesis. The manner by which they proposed to circumvent this problem was to perform a "pre-analysis" in which the speech signal was broken down into distinctive features. This would be the equivalent, in our stencil analogy, of grouping letters by visual features. For example, we can break letters down into a group that is formed with a round circle or part of a small round circle. The letters b,d,c,e,g,o,p,q, would fit into this group. (In the next chapter we will treat distinctive features like these for speech in much greater detail.)

Template Matching

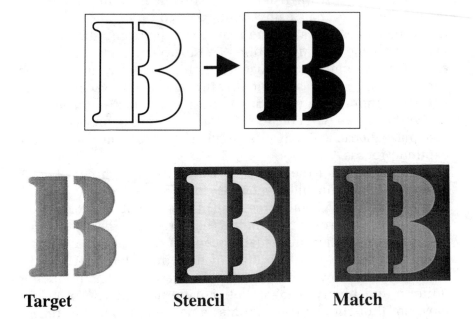

Figure 6–1. Schematic of using a stencil to illustrate the process of template matching.

An acoustic form of this visual template-matching may prove to be a useful construct for explaining speech perception. How might this template-matching procedure work in speech perception? In Figure 6–2, there is an example of a target spectra for an /i/ vowel. Below the target is an example of a very precise or restrictive template for a /i/ vowel, as well as an example of a much more general template. We can see that the restrictive template is only going to match with a very particular acoustic spectrum, whereas the more general template is going to match with a much greater variety of acoustic signals. We will return to this concept of template matching in Chapter 8 on the Theory of Acoustic Invariance, another account of speech perception. Before we discuss the theory of acoustic invariance, it will be necessary to consider distinctive features and phonetic feature detectors in the next chapter.

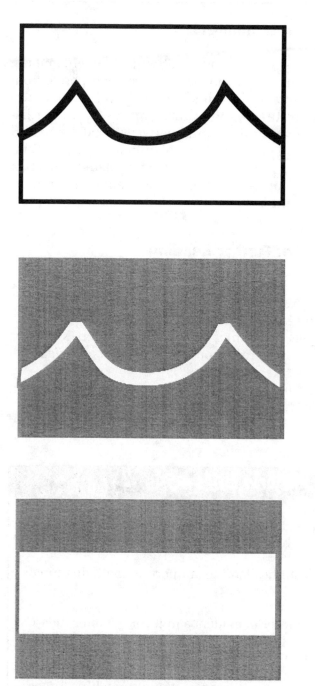

Target Spectrum

Narrow Specific Template

Wide General Template

Figure 6–2. Schematic of a target spectrum with a narrow template and a wide template which "match" the spectrum.

Summary

Motor theory represents one important attempt to overcome the problem of acoustic invariance and explain speech perception. There is evidence for and against this theory. Even if motor commands do not turn out the be the primary means by which listeners decode speech, an intimate link between production and perception is a fundamental property of human speech. Template matching, a concept borrowed from the related theory of analysis-by-synthesis, represents a useful metaphor for understanding speech perception.

For Further Reading

Borden, G., Harris, K., & Raphael, L. (1994). *Speech Science Primer: Physiology, Acoustics, and Perception of Speech* (3rd edition). Baltimore, MD: Williams & Wilkins.

Liberman, A., Cooper, F., Shankweiler, D., & Studdert-Kennedy, M. (1967). Perception of the speech code. *Psychological Review, 74*, 431–461.

Liberman, A., & Mattingly, I. (1985). The motor theory of speech perception revised. *Cognition, 21*, 1–36.

REVIEW QUESTIONS

1. What does this chapter take to be the major difficulty with the motor theory of speech perception?

2. Did early EMG studies tend to support or contradict motor theory?

3. What are some pieces of evidence in favor of motor theory?

4. How is analysis-by-synthesis different from motor theory?

5. What is a drawback to using a stencil-matching procedure to discover which letter was produced?

CHAPTER

7

Distinctive Features and Phonetic Feature Detectors

LEARNING OBJECTIVES

The concept of minimal binary distinctive acoustic features is discussed in this chapter, as well as their relationship to information theory. One goal of this chapter is to prepare the reader for understanding the theory of acoustic invariance presented in the next chapter.

The concept of phonetic feature detectors is also considered in this chapter. While there is considerable experimental evidence for their existence, which is summarized in the chapter, they remain to be isolated in the human brain.

Distinctive Features

You may already be familiar with phonological or phonetic features that are used to classify speech sounds. A matrix of these features was used to describe the various consonants of English in Figure 1–2 in Chapter 1. We also touched on the concept of features when we spoke about place-of-articulation and voicing. Probably the features that you know are articulatory-phonetic in nature. That is, they describe speech in terms of the articulatory gestures that are required to produce them. For example, you'll recall that /p/ and /b/ have a *bilabial* place of articulation because they are produced with the two (bi) lips (labial), /t/ and /d/ have an *alveolar* place of articulation because the tongue tip touches the alveolar ridge when they are produced, and /k/ and /g/ are *velar* since the tongue back makes contact with the velum. (A somewhat more precise description would be to also include the activity of the tongue—so alveolars would be *apico-alveolar* and velar sounds would be classified as *dorso-velar*.) You will also remember that it is *voicing* that distinguishes /p/ from /b/, /t/ from /d/, and /k/ from /g/. In other words, /p/ and /b/ are only different from one another in the voicing feature; otherwise, they are articulated in a similar manner.

Such a feature classification has proven useful in describing speech and its articulation. However, the qualifier *distinctive* feature has a somewhat more limited meaning. In the strictest sense of the term, distinctive features are the absolute minimal contrasts between phonemes in a language. This binary sense of the term can be traced back to the Russian linguists N. Trubetzkoy and R. Jakobson.

After Roman Jakobson emigrated to the United States after World War II, he attempted to define a set of *universal* distinctive features and the underlying acoustic property that accounted for each particular distinction. The result of this work, undertaken in collaboration with his colleagues Gunnar Fant and Morris Halle, was a monograph first published in the early 1950s entitled "Preliminaries to Speech Analysis: The Distinctive Features" (Jakobson, Fant, & Halle, 1963). What should be emphasized about the features proposed in this work is that they were intended to be universal. In other words, they were intended to be applicable, with minor adjustments, for every language. They were strictly acoustic in nature and not based on articulation.

Additionally, these features were also binary (i.e., + or –), distinctive and minimal—representing the relevant contrasts between phonemes with the fewest possible number of features.

These characteristics of Jakobson, Fant, and Halle's features are pointed out here because students are often more familiar with the set of phonological features developed by Chomsky and Halle in 1968 for the English language presented in their book *The Sound Pattern of English*. Chomsky and Halle's features were developed specifically for the English language and not intended to be universal. They are a mixture of phonological and articulatory features.

There is a special sense of distinctive employed by Jakobson, Fant, and Halle that comes from *information theory*. That is, distinctive features are optimal—they convey the minimal number of contrasts necessary. In this strict sense of distinctive, there is a mathematical formula that accounts for the minimal number of binary contrasts necessary to convey a particular piece of information. This formula is 2 to the *nth* power, where *n* equals the number of binary features. For example, if we wish to specify three places of articulation (bilabial, alveolar, and velar) we should only require two features. According to this formula, two features would allow for four contrasts (2 to the 2nd power, or $2^2 = 2 \times 2 = 4$). Thus, three terms for place-of-articulation are not distinctive and minimal because they would allow for eight contrasts! (2 to the 3rd power, or $2^3 = 2 \times 2 \times 2 = 8$). This is a rather long way of stating that the descriptive terms bilabial, alveolar, and velar are in no way minimal distinctive features.

In the features of Jakobson, Fant, and Halle the three places of articulation are handled by two binary features *compact-diffuse* and *acute-grave*. Each feature is like a polar opposite, like black and white, up and down and so forth—the presence of one attribute automatically implies the absence of its opposite. Therefore, one of the attributes is usually used for the feature and given a + or a – sign to denote its presence or absence.

The acoustic features *compact* and *acute* relate to place-of-articulation in English in the following manner. There is only one place-of-articulation that is [+ compact] (or [–diffuse]) in English, and that is the velars. Both bilabials and alveolars are [–compact] (or [+ diffuse]), so this is where the second feature acute-grave comes into play. Alveolars are [+acute] ([–grave]) whereas bilabials are [–acute] ([+grave]). We don't need to specify whether velars are acute or grave, since in English there are no contrasts between consonants that are [+ compact]. In other words, the feature [+ compact] is redundant for the feature acute-grave.

We will return to these acoustic features in Chapter 8 where we will specify to just what property of the acoustic signal they refer. Let us now consider the use of features in speech perception. Perhaps you will recall from Chapter 6, we discussed template matching in the section Analysis-by-Synthesis. There, it was pointed out that one problem with employing a template-matching procedure for speech recognition would be that listeners would have to go through the entire set of templates each time they attempt to make a match. This would be necessary to ensure that they had found the best match possible. It was also pointed out that one way of reducing the time it would take would be to make a preliminary classification by features. In other words, a feature analysis is one means of coping with the extraordinary amount of variation found in the acoustic signal of speech. A feature analysis breaks down the signal in terms of its relevant acoustic properties. Only those contrasts that are relevant for speech perception are retained, while other contrasts irrelevant to speech perception are ignored.

For example, one kind of acoustic contrast that would be ignored after a feature analysis would be differences due to speech being produced by different speakers. As we pointed out in the discussion on vowel normalization in Chapter 3, the difference between a vowel produced by an adult and one produced by a child must be ignored in speech perception. This is one example of the type of variation that would be ignored after speech was broken down by features.

Some direct evidence that listeners classify speech sounds by features comes from a classic study by Miller and Nicely (1955). In this study listeners were presented with CV (consonant-vowel) syllables in the presence of noise. With noise added, as you well know, speech is more difficult to understand. But the listening errors in Miller and Nicely's study were not random, as you might have expected. Listeners' errors were highly organized. Only certain sounds were confused for others. In fact the pattern of results from this study were organized by features. Sounds such as /p/, /t/, and /k/ that differ only by place-of-articulation features were highly confused. Voicing errors (e.g., hearing *pig* for *big*) were also common.

Another source of evidence that human speech is organized in terms of such features comes from speech errors or so-called slips of the tongue. These errors can often be explained in terms of a change in a single feature, and they are not the result of some random substitution of one speech sound for another (Fromkin, 1971, 1973).

Although we have gone into some detail here on features, it will be useful in understanding the theory of acoustic invariance in Chapter 8. As you will see, this theory is a direct extension of Jakobson, Fant, and Halle's pioneering work on a set of universal acoustic features. We will now turn our attention to phonetic feature detectors, which are an extension of phonetic features.

Phonetic Feature Detectors

Phonetic feature detectors (alternatively, linguistic feature detectors, feature analyzers, neural feature detectors) are a theoretical construct employed to help explain speech perception. Although there is a fair amount of experimental evidence for their existence, which we will briefly review in this chapter, they remain a theoretical construct. That is, no one has yet isolated phonetic feature detectors in the human brain—despite the fact that some even call them "neural" feature detectors. However, scientists have isolated neural centers sensitive to certain acoustic properties in the cat and other animals (Whitfield & Evans, 1965).

Such direct physiological research on neural feature detectors has not been undertaken on human beings, for obvious ethical reasons. (Most people don't take kindly to having electrodes placed in their brain.) Thus far, neural centers have not been isolated that respond to speech per se in the same specific manner that would be expected from a phonetic feature detector. Yet, there is a great deal of progress in this area of understanding the neural underpinnings of speech and language. Perhaps neural detectors for specific attributes of the speech signal will be isolated before long.

In any case, the aim of the remainder of this chapter is to review the experimental evidence for phonetic feature detectors, and discuss why they are useful theoretical constructs for explaining speech perception.

The main source of evidence for phonetic feature detectors comes from the *selective adaptation* procedure. In selective adaptation, a certain acoustic property detector is "fatigued" through repeated presentation of auditory stimuli with that acoustic property present. For example, Eimas and Corbit (1973) investigated the voicing contrast. They found that either the voiced or the voiceless member of a pair (such as *b* and *p*) could be adapted by repeated auditory presentations (typically more than a hundred) of its voicing opposite. In other words, after repeated presentations of a voiced sound, listeners hear more stimuli as voiceless.

First of all, these investigators obtained identification functions for a continuum of stimuli that differed only in VOT (voice onset time). They then demonstrated that the identification function for a particular subject could be shifted or displaced after exposure to repeated exemplars of a stimulus. The adaptation effect is largest for stimuli that are near the original phonetic boundary.

If *ba*, for example, was the adapting stimulus that was repeated over and over, then the identification function shifted in the direction away from the voicing end of the continuum and the subject "heard" more voiceless tokens. This shift takes place presumably because the voicing detector is fatigued, and it becomes more difficult to make this detector react to voicing. The result is that there are more voiceless stops perceived. Adaptation then, shifts the perceptual boundary point toward the adapting stimulus, resulting in more stimuli being heard as the voicing opposite. Figure 7–1 is a representation of this adaptation shift.

The adaptation effect is not only seen in identification, but also in discrimination functions. Such neural property detectors appear to be centrally based and not part of the peripheral nervous system. This is because the adaptation effect also occurs when the adapting stimulus and the stimuli to be identified are presented in opposite ears (Eimas, Cooper, & Corbit, 1973). If feature detectors were peripherally based, the adapting stimulus would have to be presented to the same ear as the identification stimuli.

It should be pointed out that not all researchers are entirely comfortable with such a straightforward mapping from the acoustic signal to neural property detectors and there is some controversy in this area. In spite of this, neural property detectors continue to be a useful construct in explaining human speech perception.

Phonetic feature detectors seem to be specific to speech. When the vowel portion of the adapting stimulus is removed, such that only the formant transition portion of the initial con-

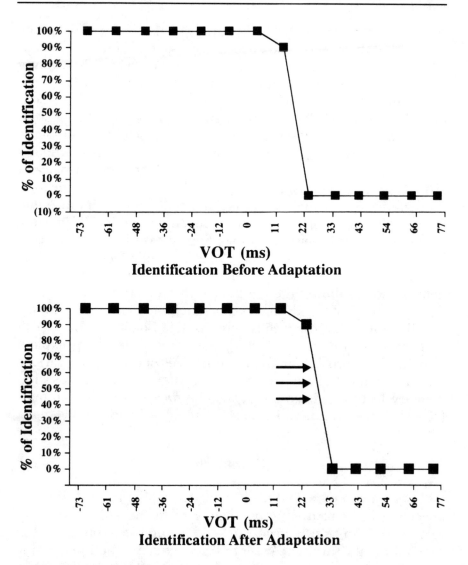

Figure 7–1. Illustration of the adaptation effect of repeated presentations of an initial voiced stop on a voice-voiceless identification function. Identification shifts away from the adaptation stimulus—in this case towards more voiceless identifications.

sonant remains, there is significantly less adaptation. (You will recall from Chapter 4 on consonant perception, that without the vowel portion of the syllable, the remaining portion does not sound like a consonant and is typically not even recognized as speech.) Eimas et al. (1973) hypothesize that feature detectors "are part of the specialized speech processor, inasmuch as adaptation of a voicing detector . . . occurred only when the voicing information was presented in a speech context" (p. 247).

Features have not only been investigated for the voicing contrast, but also for place-of-articulation (Cooper, 1974). Another important aspect of the phonetic feature detector for voicing is that apparently it operates independently of place-of-articulation. In other words, the voiced stop *d* (with an alveolar place of articulation) was nearly as effective in changing the identification function for *b* - *p* as was the bilabial *b*. This in turn implies that feature detectors work at the phonetic (or feature) level. Thus the voicing detector is sensitive to voicing across different places of articulation. It is not individual b-p, d-t, g-k voicing detectors that are involved here, but there seems to be a single general voicing detector across these different places of articulation.

Phonetic feature detectors may help explain the extreme rapidity with which speech is perceived. In Chapter 11 on speech perception in infants, feature detectors may also help explain how the newborn infant already organizes speech along various relevant parameters such as the voicing dimension. Perhaps rudimentary feature detectors may also be present in other animals (speech perception in animals is the topic of Chapter 13).

Summary

Although a variety of feature systems are available for describing speech, minimal distinctive acoustic features have a very restricted definition. The goal of such features is to break speech down into its minimal essential acoustic distinctions. Using such features, the 40-some phonemes of American English could be broken down into approximately 7 binary contrasts. This would greatly reduce the task of processing speech for perception. Acoustic features also imply that the information required to distinguish the sounds of speech is directly available in the acoustic signal of speech.

The concept of phonetic feature detectors is an outgrowth of feature theory. Phonetic feature detectors imply that there is a specific neural substrate devoted to detecting of the presence or absence of each particular phonetic contrast. If we combine these two notions—one, that speech can be broken down into minimal essential sound contrasts and two, that there are neural detectors that react specifically to the absence or presence of these same acoustic properties—we begin to get a clearer picture of how speech perception might occur.

For Further Reading

Cooper, W., (1974). Adaptation of phonetic feature analyzers for place of articulation. *Journal of the Acoustical Society of America, 56,* 617–627.

Eimas, P., (1974). Auditory and linguistic processing of cues for place of articulation by infants. *Perception and Psychophysics, 16,* 513–521.

Eimas, P., Cooper, W., & Corbit, J., (1973). Some properties of linguistic feature detectors. *Perception and Psychophysics, 13,* 247–252.

Eimas, P., & Corbit, J., (1973). Selective adaptation of linguistic feature detectors. *Perception and Psychophysics, 4,* 99–109.

Eimas, P., & Miller, J., (1978). Effects of selective adaptation on the perception of speech and visual forms: Evidence for feature detectors. In R. D. Walk and H. L. Pick Jr. (Eds.), *Perception and Experience.* New York: Plenum.

Jakobson, R., Fant, G., & Halle, M. (1963). *Preliminaries to Speech Analysis: The Distinctive Features.* Cambridge, MA: MIT Press. (Original work published in 1952)

REVIEW QUESTIONS

1. Explain why it is impossible for the terms *bilabial, alveolar* and *velar* to represent minimal distinctive features for place-of-articulation of the stop consonants in English. (Hint: Count the number of terms and compare it to the number of place-of-articulation contrasts in English.)

2. If the three terms above **were** minimal distinctive features, how many place-of-articulation contrasts could they distinguish?

(continued)

(continued)

3. How do we know that listeners do organize speech into features?

4. What is the main source of evidence for the existence of phonetic feature detectors?

5. Have phonetic feature detectors for speech been isolated in the human brain?

6. What would be the advantage of having phonetic feature detectors?

C H A P T E R

8

A Theory of
Acoustic Invariance

LEARNING OBJECTIVES

Readers are acquainted with the basic premises of the theory of acoustic invariance. Building on material presented in previous chapters, acoustic invariance is also placed within its historical context. The goal is this chapter is to present the basic concepts of acoustic invariance as simply as possible. The reader should gain an overall picture of acoustic invariance and have some idea of its development, but also understand how it differs from previous theories. Work related to acoustic invariance is also considered. This material is required for a modern treatment of speech perception. The widespread attention given to this theory suggests that it represents the most significant development in our understanding of speech perception since motor theory.

Acoustic Invariance

You will recall the problem of acoustic invariance from Chapter 4 on the perception of consonants. We have already discussed several solutions that have been proposed for this problem—especially locus theory and the motor theory. In this chapter, we will discuss a more recent proposal that extends directly from the work of Roman Jakobson and his colleagues on acoustic features presented in Chapter 7. This theory was named the theory of acoustic invariance by its developers—Professors Kenneth Stevens and Sheila Blumstein.

When we discussed the problem of invariance for place-of-articulation for stop consonants, you will recall that we did not completely discard the possibility that invariance might still be found in the acoustic signal itself. As was already mentioned, even the advocates of motor theory did not deny this possibility: they were simply more optimistic that a solution would be found in terms of speech production.

The theory of acoustic invariance is essentially based on this alternative that invariance is to be found directly in the acoustic signal. Thus, in some ways, it can be considered as a step back in time, in the sense that it looks at the acoustic signal itself as the source of invariance—just as researchers had proposed before the elaboration of a motor theory. In this chapter, we will try to specify just what aspect of the acoustic signal that Stevens and Blumstein propose carries invariant cues for place-of-articulation.

Before we do so, it will be useful to briefly review the information on vowel perception that was presented in Chapter 3. You will recall there was evidence that the ear is capable of formant extraction via a Fourier analysis—a rudimentary form of spectrographic representation. Therefore this much of the "machinery" for a theory of acoustic invariance is already required to explain vowel perception. In the theory of acoustic invariance, a similar type of spectral analysis (using linear predictive coding or LPC) is directed to the acoustic signal for consonants as well. However, this analysis is applied at one specific point in the consonant signal—at the burst resulting from the release of the consonant obstruction from the lips.

The theory postulates that there is sufficient information in the acoustic signal at the release of the consonant (and up to some 20 ms afterwards) to specify uniquely its place-of-articulation. It is important to point out that, even if the theory depends on some portion of the signal after the burst, we are not yet talking about the entire formant transitions (which are traditionally considered to be quite a bit longer, at least some 50 ms). At 20 ms and shorter, in most instances the acoustic signal will not yet be into the formant structure portion of the speech signal; therefore, there would be no transitions.

Once a formant extraction analysis has been applied to the signal, it is categorized along the acoustic features for place-of-articulation hypothesized by Jakobson and his colleagues. The innovation with the theory of acoustic invariance is that Stevens and Blumstein have given a precise definition to the hypothetical acoustic features first proposed by Jakobson and colleagues. In the theory of acoustic invariance, the acoustic spectrum at the point of release is *compact* if there is one formant peak that predominates. Figure 8–1 gives an example of a compact spectrum. If the determination is + compact, this spectrum is from the velar place-of-articulation. It is not necessary to characterize further whether or not it is acute or grave since there is no acute-grave distinction in English for consonants that are compact.

If the spectrum is not compact, then it is considered *diffuse*. The spectrum is then further analyzed as to whether or not it is *acute* or *grave*. If the formant peaks are rising in amplitude as a function of frequency then the spectrum is considered acute and the determination for place-of-articulation is alveolar. If the formant peaks are falling the spectrum is considered grave and the signal is considered to have come from a bilabial place-of-articulation. (See Figure 8–1.)

Although we have just described the postulates of Stevens and Blumstein's theory, we have not completely described the theory. This is because in their theory of acoustic invariance, Blumstein and Stevens (1979) make use of a template-matching procedure. You will recall template-matching from our discussion of analysis-by-synthesis in Chapter 6 on motor theory. These researchers proposed that the determination of place-of-articulation could proceed by means of the fitting of the signal to acoustic templates.

Static Versus Dynamic Cues

It is important to note that the information used to determine place-of-articulation in Stevens and Blumstein's theory is *static*,

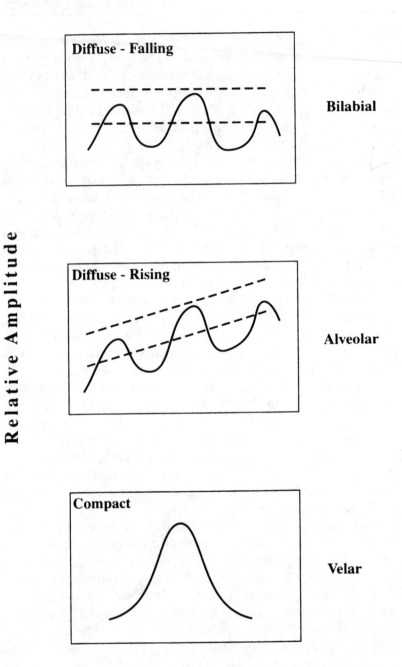

Figure 8–1. Spectral templates for places of articulation in English. (Adapted with permission from Blumstein & Stevens [1979]. Acoustic Invariance in Speech Production: Evidence From Measurements of the Spectral Characteristics of Stop Consonants. *Journal of the Acoustical Society of America, 66*(4), 1001–1017. Copyright 1979 by the American Institute of Physics.)

in the sense that we are only considering the acoustic signal at one particular fixed point in time. Weaker versions of acoustic invariance developed by Kewley-Port (1983) and Forrest, Weismer, Milenkovic, and Dougall (1988) utilize information gathered *dynamically* over a longer time frame. These dynamic versions propose that successive slices of the signal are necessary to specify the invariance for place-of-articulation. Although Stevens and Blumstein's account of invariance is not incompatible with dynamic information also being utilized, their theory is stronger in that it proposes that dynamic information is not necessary, and that the invariance can be specified with acoustic information from one particular point in time.

Note that Stevens and Blumstein's theory does not postulate additional machinery to determine place-of-articulation. In other words, the spectral analysis on which it relies is already necessary to explain vowel perception. In this sense, their theory is *parsimonious*—it uses the same mechanisms or theoretical constructs that are already required to explain vowel perception. The only additions are: (a) the proviso that the spectral analysis is directed at a particular portion of the signal (i.e., at the burst resulting from the release of the consonant) and (b) there is a classification of the resulting spectrum by means of specific attributes or features (i.e., templates that specify the acoustic features for place-of-articulation).

To test the predictions of their theory Stevens and Blumstein categorized 1800 natural speech CV syllable productions according to place-of-articulation, without knowing what speech had been produced. They found that their classifications for place-of-articulation were about 85% accurate for initial stop consonants, although somewhat less accurate for stop consonants in the syllable final position (Blumstein & Stevens, 1979).

Some Additional Comments

Some additional comments on acoustic invariance are in order to avoid potential misunderstandings. Although Stevens and Blumstein feel that the spectrum specified at the release of the consonant provides sufficient information to determine place-of-articulation, they do *not* entirely discount the potential contribution of additional cues such as formant transitions. Thus the shape of the spectrum at the moment of consonant release may not be the *only* source of information for making the determination of place-of-articulation. What the proponents of acoustic invariance were seeking was the *minimal* amount of information required to determine place- of-articulation. In other words, these researchers sought to formulate the strongest theory possible. However, they do not deny the potential contribution of other sources of information such as formant transitions. As these researchers state:

> The results of the vowel context analyses indicated that the acoustic characteristics of the vowel environments do have an effect on the classification of the appropriate place of articulation. Nevertheless, this vowel dependency is in a much more limited sense than, for example, the vowel context effects found in the perception of various attributes of the acoustic signal, such as burst frequency and transition motions. (Blumstein & Stevens 1979, p. 1011)

Repp (1988) has proposed one potential means of integrating these two sources of information (one from the shape of the spectrum at consonantal release, the other from formant transitions). He theorizes that the release of the consonant may, via the theory of acoustic invariance, provide a static snapshot view of what the articulators are doing at the moment of the release of the consonant. As Repp states: "According to acoustic theory, the spectrum of the transient should contain peaks reflecting the vocal tract resonances immediately after the release. Since the excitation is so brief and uniform, the transient provides essentially an acoustic snapshot of the vocal tract" (p. 380). Formant transitions could then provide additional dynamic information. If these two sources of cues provide similar information for place-of-articulation, then the perceptual task may be easier than in cases where the two sources of information are in conflict. It may be the case that these different sources of information are used to different degrees according to the particular perceptual situation.

It is clear that despite the potential breakthrough provided by the theory of acoustic invariance, more research is needed in this area. This chapter has served to outline the acoustic invariance proposal that has gained an increasing number of adherents since it was first proposed over a decade ago.

There have been some preliminary attempts to investigate acoustic invariance in speakers with speech disorders (e.g., adult aphasia: Shinn & Blumstein, 1983; children with hearing impairment: Ryalls, Baum, & Larouche, 1991). It is expected that more research within this theoretical framework will further our understanding of both normal and disordered speech.

Summary

The theory of acoustic invariance proposes that the information required for perception of place-of-articulation can be found directly within the acoustic signal. The work of Stevens and Blumstein provides a precise definition for the acoustic features first proposed by Jakobson and colleagues in the 1950s. These researchers have also provided a test of the accuracy of their spectral features in classifying real speech data, using a template-matching procedure. The broad consideration given this theory in the contemporary specialized scientific literature on speech perception suggests that it may already have gained wider acceptance than motor theory.

For Further Reading

Blumstein, S. (1986). On acoustic invariance in speech. In J. Perkell & D. Klatt (Eds.), *Invariance and Variability in Speech Processes*. Hillsdale, NJ: Erlbaum.

Blumstein, S., & Stevens, K. (1979). Acoustic invariance in speech production: Evidence from measurements of the spectral characteristics of stop consonants. *Journal of the Acoustical Society of America, 66*(4), 1001–1017.

Blumstein, S., & Stevens, K. (1980). Perceptual invariance and onset spectra for stop consonants in different vowel environments. *Journal of the Acoustical Society of America, 67*(2), 648–662.

Blumstein, S., & Stevens, K. (1981). Phonetic features and acoustic invariance for speech. *Cognition, 10*, 25–32.

Stevens, K., & Blumstein, S. (1981). The search for invariant acoustic correlates of phonetic features. In P. Eimas & J. Miller (Eds.), *Perspectives on the Study of Speech* (pp. 1–38). Hillsdale, NJ: Erlbaum.

REVIEW QUESTIONS

1. How does acoustic invariance describe the spectrum for the velar place-of-articulation?

2. Does the use of spectral information over successive periods of time represent a stronger or a weaker version of acoustic invariance?

3. Approximately how accurate were Blumstein and Stevens (1979) in classifying speech data for the place-of-articulation of initial stop consonants?

4. Do Stevens and Blumstein completely rule out the potential contribution of formant transitions in determining place-of-articulation?

5. Why is it important to consider the acoustic information provided in the burst? (In other words, what is the advantage of the spectral information from this particular point in time?)

CHAPTER

9

Dichotic Listening

LEARNING OBJECTIVES

Readers will learn the basic principles involved in dichotic listening as well as its physiological bases. Differences between vowels and consonants for dichotic listening are discussed. These differences help us better understand the differences between vowel and consonant speech perception. Since it differs from speech, the processing of music is also briefly treated.

Ear Differences for Speech

You may have noticed that people often dial the telephone with the phone resting on the left ear and then change ears when someone answers on the other end. Perhaps you do this and you never noticed consciously. Or maybe you have observed other people doing this, although you don't do it yourself. In any case, many people do this and perhaps you are wondering why any-one would do so. One potential answer could be because of the *dichotic listening* effect.

What is dichotic listening? Essentially, it refers to any situa-tion in which different sounds are presented to the two ears. If two different and competing acoustic signals are delivered to each of the ears at the same time, generally the right ear does a better job of reporting verbal stimuli. This is because, although both ears are connected to each side of the brain, there are usu-ally somewhat stronger contralateral connections (i.e., right ear to left hemisphere of the brain, or left ear to right hemisphere) than there are ipsilateral connections (i.e., right ear to the right hemisphere of the brain, or left ear to left hemisphere). Since the left hemisphere is more specialized for treatment of at least some forms of verbal stimuli, then subjects are usually somewhat more accurate at reporting what words they heard with their right ear than what they heard with their left ear.

The dichotic listening procedure was first developed by Broadbent (1954), who used spoken digits. The dichotic tech-nique was then further developed by Kimura (1961), who also offered a neurological explanation for the dichotic effect. Her ex-planation still seems to be the most popular one today (although there are some alternative explanations such as from Geffen and Quinn, 1984). In Kimura's (1967) own words:

> The explanation for the right-ear superiority on the digits test then, was that the right ear had better connections with the left hemisphere than did the left ear, and since the left hemisphere was the one in which speech sounds were presumably analyzed, the right-ear sounds had the advantage of having better access to these speech centres (p. 164)

Two points are worth emphasizing here. First of all, each ear is connected to each hemisphere. No one should get the idea that each ear is *only* connected to the opposite hemisphere. It is sim-ply the case that there are usually somewhat more fibers (or larg-er connections) between the ear and the *opposite* hemisphere, than there are between the ear and the hemisphere on the same side. This typical situation is represented in Figure 9–1A (repro-duced from Sidtis, 1982).

But there also seems to be a significant amount of variation from individual to individual. Other nontypical forms of rela-

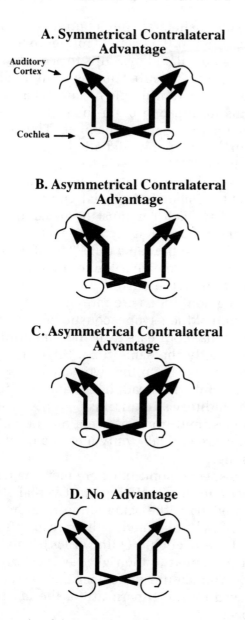

A. Symmetrical Contralateral Advantage

Auditory Cortex

Cochlea

B. Asymmetrical Contralateral Advantage

C. Asymmetrical Contralateral Advantage

D. No Advantage

Figure 9–1. Schematic of the various potential ear-brain connection relationships. Bolder arrows represent stronger neural connections, lighter arrows weaker neural connections. (Adapted with permission from Sidtis [1982]. Predicting Brain Organization From Dichotic Listening Performance: Cortical and Subcortical Functional Asymmetries Contribute to Perceptual Asymmetries. *Brain and Language, 17,* 287–300. Copyright 1982 by Academic Press.)

tionship between ipsilateral and contralateral auditory pathways are represented in B, C, and D in Figure 9–1. These different situations are postulated by Sidtis to account for some of the differences in dichotic listening among individuals on the same task. However, the basic principle of somewhat better contralateral connections from ear to brain than ipsilateral connections seems to hold up in a general manner. The basic theoretical assumptions underlying the dichotic model are reviewed in Geffen and Quinn (1984).

Second, it should be pointed out that the dichotic effect occurs only under somewhat special conditions. The acoustic signals delivered to each ear must be in competition—that is, they must be of similar intensity and length and they must be delivered to each ear at the same time. The effect is not the same when one channel is somewhat louder than the other, or if one stimulus is longer than the other. It is for these reasons that true dichotic listening conditions are rare, if not nonexistent, in the real world outside of the psychoacoustic laboratory. Under most listening conditions, both ears hear the same thing, though not necessarily at exactly the same time. Slight differences in the timing of auditory signals to the two ears are used in the localization of sound. But with headphones and computer-controlled presentation of auditory stimuli, it is possible to deliver the conflicting auditory stimuli that induce a dichotic effect. However these conditions are typically only met in a carefully controlled laboratory setting.

When these special conditions are met, the right ear is typically more accurate in identifying most verbal stimuli than the left ear presented with the same stimuli, (although ear effects can also sometimes be obtained without respecting each of these dichotic conditions; Geffen & Quinn, 1984). This greater accuracy for stimuli presented to the right ear is referred to as a *right ear advantage*. You should remember that the advantage of the *right* ear is based on the superiority of the *left* hemisphere for processing speech.

How do we know that the dichotic effect is really due to the left hemisphere's specialization for speech? Well, for one thing, we know that people usually become aphasic (or have severe speech and language problems) much more often as a result of neurological insult to the left hemisphere than as a result of damage to the right hemisphere.

There are also electrophysiological studies, and other techniques such as the PET (positive emission tomography) scan, which demonstrate greater activity associated with processing verbal stimuli in the left side of the brain than on the right. In other words, there are other independent sources of evidence for the superiority of the left hemisphere for processing verbal stimuli.

Consonant Vowel Differences

Some additional comments here concern the nature of the verbal stimuli. In the earliest experiments using dichotic listening, there was a clear and statistically significant advantage only for stop consonants in CV (consonant-vowel) syllables (Shankweiler & Studdert-Kennedy, 1967). In other words, similar to categorical perception, there seems to be a difference between consonants and vowels for dichotic listening.

Although ear effects for vowels are not clear, there are conditions under which right ear advantages are elicited for vowel stimuli (Divenyi & Effron, 1979; Haggard, 1971). In a general manner, manipulations that increase the difficulty of the perceptual task seem to increase the right ear advantage for vowels. If vowels are presented with noise, or if the differences between the vowels are reduced, the right ear advantage becomes stronger (Divenyi & Effron, 1979). However, overall results are not very clear for vowels. The ear advantage for vowels is also much less reliable than the one found for consonants (Blumstein, Goodglass, & Tarter, 1975). Some studies have found a left ear advantage for vowel stimuli (in other words, the right hemisphere is better at processing vowels).

We won't concern ourselves further with the exact nature of the ear advantage for vowels. What is important to consider is that it is very different from the consistent and rather strong advantage of the right ear that is typically found for stop consonants. Further discussion attempting to account for the correlation between findings for categorical perception and dichotic listening can be found in Ryalls (1987b).

Speech Versus Music

It is important to consider that, in complement to the superiority of the left hemisphere for certain types of speech stimuli, the right hemisphere seems to be somewhat better than the left for certain types of musical signals. In other words, certain forms of musical stimuli are better processed by the *left* ear, because the *right* hemisphere seems to be better at processing these stimuli.

From more recent work, we now know that the musical competence of the listener must also be taken into consideration. If the listener is more of an expert musician it appears that it is the *left* hemisphere that is better at processing music. (One interpretation of this effect is that music becomes a kind of language for music experts. Expert musicians can associate verbal labels with musical stimuli. Hence, musical stimuli are processed in the left hemisphere for such listeners.)

We now understand that it is important to know the exact nature of the listening task that listeners are required to perform. When non-musically trained subjects are asked to listen for differences in short melodies, they naturally are somewhat better at doing so with the stimuli that is presented to their *left* ears.

However, when the same subjects are required to pay attention to the discrete local changes in the melodies, their ear advantage shifts to the *right* ear (Peretz, Morais, & Bertelson 1987). In other words, not only must we consider the nature of the stimuli (musical versus verbal; consonant versus vowel), and the type of subject (musically sophisticated or not), we also have to consider what exact task listeners are instructed to perform.

Right Brain, Left Brain, Whole Brain

Recently the popular media has rather grossly exaggerated this concept of hemispheric differences. There are now manuals that purport to teach us how to better exploit our supposedly underused right hemispheres, or how we can foster better communication between our left and right brains. Most of the original experiments on which a lot of this reasoning is based typically only demonstrated *slight* differences, which have been somewhat exaggerated in the popular literature.

It is not as if we are completely deaf to speech stimuli that is presented to the left ear. (We know this is patently not the case, because there are plenty of people who perceive speech perfectly well who are completely deaf in their left ears, for example.) Nor is it true that the right hemisphere is not capable of any processing of speech material. It has been shown that the right hemisphere seems to be somewhat better at processing intonation—the more melodic or musiclike aspects of speech (Blumstein & Cooper, 1974).

In any case, it is useful to remember that the two halves of the brain already communicate with each other. Not only is there the important link provided by the corpus callosum, which connects the two hemispheres, but the two hemispheres are also connected at their bases and share many common subcortical structures. There are also connections provided through longer U-shaped fibers.

Although it may be popular to emphasize the *differences* between the two hemispheres at the present time, this is probably only because we thought of the two hemispheres as exactly the same for so long. There are certainly no indications of these differences that can be observed from visually inspecting the two hemispheres of the brain.

In the long run, the pendulum will probably eventually swing back in the other direction, and the holistic or ultimately joint nature of the two hemispheres of the brain will probably tend once again to be emphasized. In the final analysis, the entire brain works together as a whole, and it may be somewhat artificial to compartmentalize different aspects of what the brain does. Some apparent differences may occur only under artificial laboratory conditions. Such differences may turn out to be a poor representation of what actually occurs in the brain in everyday functioning. Perhaps it is more useful to emphasize the manner in which the brain works together as a whole, rather than the manner in which the two halves work independently.

Summary

Dichotic listening reveals that vowels and consonants recruit somewhat different speech processing areas in the brain. The dichotic listening paradigm is one of the important ways in which differences between the two hemispheres of the brain have been studied. Typically, the left hemisphere is better at processing verbal material.

While the popular media have seized upon these differences between the two halves of the brain in order to promote the notion of two independently functioning systems, it should be emphasized that both contribute to language processing in an integrated manner.

For Further Reading

Geffen, G., & Quinn, K. (1984). Hemispheric specialization and ear advantages in processing speech. *Psychological Bulletin, 96*(2), 273–291.

Kimura, D. (1967). Functional asymmetry of the brain in dichotic listening. *Cortex, 3*, 163–168.

Peretz, I., Morais, J., & Bertelson, P. (1987). Shifting ear differences in melody recognition through strategy inducement. *Brain and Cognition, 6*, 202–215.

Shankweiler, D., & Studdert-Kennedy, M. (1967). Identification of consonants and vowels presented to left and right ears. *Quarterly Journal of Experimental Psychology, 19*, 59–63.

Sidtis, J. (1982). Predicting brain organization from dichotic listening performance: Cortical and subcortical functional asymmetries contribute to perceptual asymmetries. *Brain and Language, 17*, 287–300.

REVIEW QUESTIONS

1. Briefly explain why there is a difference in speech perception performance between the two ears.

2. Because the right ear is better at processing speech stimuli, does this mean that the right ear is connected to the left hemisphere exclusively? If not, why?

3. Do vowels and consonants result in equal ear effects? If not, what are the differences?

4. What are other sources of evidence that the two halves of the brain are specialized for speech and language differently?

5. How is the processing of music different from that for speech? Is there a difference between amateur and expert musicians?

CHAPTER

10

Parallel Distributed Processing Models: Bottom-Up Versus Top-Down

LEARNING OBJECTIVES

The goal of this chapter is to introduce the concepts of top-down, bottom-up, and parallel distributed processing. Some of the evidence for top-down processing in speech perception is presented. Parallel distributed processing models have sparked the development of neural network computers. One influential model of word recognition, the cohort model, is also discussed.

Sound and Meaning

Although only the extraction of meaning from sound is typically considered in speech perception, there are actually two sources of information brought to bear in the perception of speech. These two sources of information are referred to by the terms *bottom-up* and *top-down*. Bottom-up refers to using the acoustic information present in the speech signal to discover what word is being uttered; top-down refers to the use of pragmatic, semantic, and other forms of linguistic information in this same process. In other words, at one end of speech perception, there is the pure sound information from what we hear in speech. At the other end, we can use information such as imagining what is a possible word in the language.

While everyone is familiar with the bottom-up information that is used in speech perception (this is basically all we have talked about in this book so far), people are often less aware of the contribution of top-down information. Yet, taking one of the most well-known top-down influences on speech perception, there is ample evidence that whether or not a certain sequence of phonemes can exist as a potential word of a particular language has a powerful effect on what listeners actually hear.

Listeners are always actively seeking to make sense out of a spoken message. Under some conditions they will actually replace missing sounds in order to complete a word. There have been several studies of this effect, called *phonemic restoration*, and listeners may even remain unaware that a phoneme has been replaced by silence or noise (Samuel, 1979, 1980; Warren, 1970) when they fill in the missing phoneme to complete a whole word.

It is actually logical that people are more familiar with bottom-up rather than top-down processes, since most speech research has focused on the former instead of the latter. Only recently has research revealed the extent of the so-called top-down influences in speech perception. Perhaps it is also the case that top-down influences are somewhat less obvious, since the sound spectrograph and other devices have made the bottom-up portion of speech perception somewhat more visible. No machine yet has made the top-down influences in speech perception equally observable, except perhaps, in a very limited sense, the computer.

Computer Models

Although the computer has not really enabled us to "see" the influence of top-down processes, it has enabled us to gain a better understanding of their potential role through computer modeling of speech perception. First of all though, we should consider why we would even want a computer to be able to model human speech perception. Well, for one thing it would be much easier to talk to a computer than type to one on a keyboard. Speaking frees up one's hands to accomplish other things. Many more people are able to speak than are able to read and write. Some persons with disabilities are more capable of speaking to a computer than they are of typing on a keyboard. A final consequence is that if we could speak numbers into a telephone where they were recognized by a centralized dialing mechanism, telephone companies could save millions of dollars worth of the dialing components that are now necessary in each telephone (Lieberman, personal communication).

In any case, computer models that have attempted to duplicate human speech perception have been required to build in top-down information in order to accomplish this task. This doesn't necessarily mean that speech perception is accomplished the same way in human beings. Yet parallel research in human perception has revealed that humans do indeed use top-down information.

A very interesting development has occurred in certain contemporary computer models. While the computer has been a powerful metaphor for the human brain ever since it was first developed, a shift in the other direction has been taking place since the late 1980s. That is, for the first time in history, what scientists have learned about the brain has had an influence on computers. Computer models have been developed to simulate the neural networks of the human brain, and a new type of computer has resulted (the so-called parallel or neural network computer).

We are not going to review all of these developments here because of the magnitude and rapidly changing nature of this area of investigation. Rather, we are going to consider how these developments have changed our concept of human speech perception. To do so, we need to consider the newer computer models referred to above. These so-called neural network models are also some-times called PDP models for *Parallel Distributed Processing*. The major difference between PDP models and the older serial models is the manner in which data are processed. In traditional comput-er processing, each step must be completed before moving onto the next step. For example, the results of one calculation must be completed before the next step can begin. This type of serial pro-cessing is made explicit in a computer flow chart—one step must be accomplished before moving onto the next.

In parallel models, this constraint is circumvented and process-ing in the next stage can occur before the previous step is com-pletely accomplished. This type of parallel processing is more sim-ilar to the way the human brain apparently functions. PDP models have proven extremely popular in the field of cognitive science since they can successfully model complex human behaviors. They are especially useful in coping with the huge variation encountered in such tasks as recognizing handwriting (every individual seems to have his or her own way of writing something) or speech (each indi-vidual also has his or her own way of saying something).

If we think about the way that speech is produced, we know that the articulation of one segment is not always accomplished before the articulation of the next segment begins. For example, it is typical in English to begin opening the velo-pharyngeal port for a nasal consonant during the articulation of a preceding vowel. This results in a nasalized vowel. Since there is not a phonemic difference between nasalized and unnasalized vowels in English, it does not matter if the vowel is nasalized. This anticipation of an articulatory gesture is called *anticipatory coarticulation*. But coar-ticulation can also occur in the other direction. For example the lip-rounding gesture necessary for a rounded vowel may still be present in a consonant several phonemes later. This type of spillover, common in speech production, may also be present in speech perception. It is at least necessary that the speech percep-tual mechanism be capable of handling such spillover of acoustic information present in the speech signal.

Modeling Speech Perception

Elman and McClelland (1984) have considered the process of speech perception within a PDP framework. Figure 10–1 is a rep-resentation of how nodes at different levels interact in their

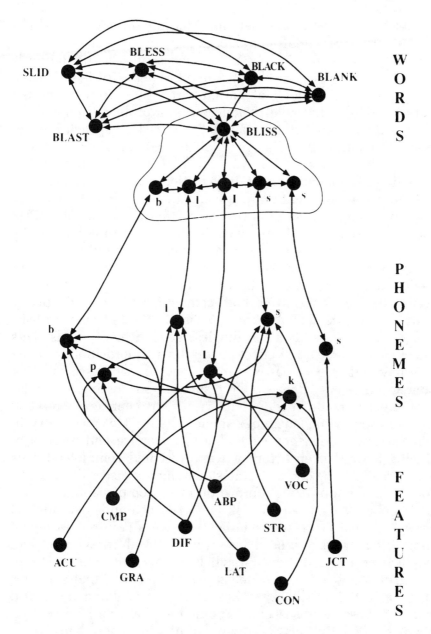

Figure 10–1. Schematic of a PDP (parallel distributed processing) model of word recognition demonstrating the interaction of nodes at different levels. (Reprinted from Elman & McClelland [1984]. Speech Perception as a Cognitive Process: The Interactive Activation Model. In N. Lass [Ed.], *Speech and Language: Advances in Basic Research and Practice* [Vol. 10]. New York: Academic Press. Copyright 1984 with permission from Academic Press.)

model. In their article, Elman and McClelland consider why it was previously difficult to model human speech perception and how a PDP model might be more successful. Coarticulation is one of the processes that they point out as being difficult to cope with in previous models of speech perception. They claim that not only does coarticulation not present a problem in a parallel model, but it may actually facilitate the task of speech perception. Elman and McClelland's article is a good review of the difficulties faced in explaining speech perception. Although it is tempting to consider each of these difficulties individually here, we will turn our attention to some of the experimental work in speech perception that contributed to the development of PDP models. Discussion of this work is also going to elucidate the nature of the top-down influence in speech perception.

Marslen-Wilson has shown that listeners are able to *shadow* (repeat what they have just heard) faster when the sentences they were asked to repeat were both semantically and syntactically well-formed (Marslen-Wilson & Welsh, 1978). Subjects are least successful with random meaningless sequences of words. This effect demonstrates the effect of top-down information. But the top-down effect becomes even more obvious when we consider some of Marslen-Wilson's other results for shadowing. He found that listeners could shadow with very short latencies, about 250 ms—or roughly the length of a single syllable. This means that in polysyllabic words they were able to **recognize and begin producing a word even before it was presented completely!** This result seems to be one of the most convincing pieces of evidence for the role of top-down information in speech perception.

Marslen-Wilson and Welsh (1978) also found that subjects would correct errors in material they were required to repeat more often when the error occurred in the third syllable than when it occurred in the first syllable. Cole and Jakimik (1978) found that subjects could detect errors faster in final syllables than in initial syllables. As Elman and McClelland point out, both of these results seem to point out that word perception involved a continuous "narrowing of possible candidates."

At the onset of a word, there are a lot of possible sounds that could follow. Since they cannot yet guess what a word is, listeners are more dependent on the acoustic information present in the signal. But as more of the word is heard, there are fewer and fewer potential candidates. In many cases, a single possibility can be determined before the word has even been entirely presented. Marslen-Wilson (1980) has claimed that words are in fact recognized at that point in time when enough information has been presented to eliminate all other possible candidates. Notice this point will be different for different words, according to how many similar words exist beginning with a similar sequence of phonemes.

What seems to occur is that bottom-up information is primary at the beginnings of words while there is practically no contribution of top-down information; but by the end of the word top-down information has become primary and there is very little contribution of the sound signal by the end of the word.

All of these experimental results have shown that not only are both bottom-up and top-down sources of information actively brought to bear in speech perception, their relative contribution varies at different parts of the word. Elman and McClelland have attempted to develop a model of speech perception that takes all of this experimental evidence into consideration. Consistent with Marslen-Wilson's claim, in their model, words are recognized when all other candidates have been eliminated.

Our goal here is not to discuss the details of any particular model, but rather to point out the important contribution of top-down information in speech perception. There is a definite clinical implication of this top-down information. For many years, it was not obvious why children with hearing impairment not only had trouble perceiving speech, but that they were also very often very poor readers as well. Recently, we have begun to understand that not only has their hearing impairment made it more difficult to gather bottom-up information from the speech signal, but children who have had poor hearing from birth also often have much less complete top-down information which they can use in speech perception.

In other words, not only do children with hearing impairment have trouble hearing which phonemes are present in the acoustic signal, they consequently also have less exposure to what are potential words in the language. Such children typically have restricted vocabularies and are less experienced in making the connection between sound and symbol. It is important that we become aware of these higher level influences in speech perception if we are to become more effective in compensating the detrimental effects of hearing loss and other disorders affecting speech perception.

Summary

The process of employing information contained in the acoustic signal to deduce meaning is referred to as bottom-up, while the influence of meaning on the perception of sound is referred to as top-down. At the onset of spoken words, perception is entirely dependent upon acoustic content, while recognition of meaning has the largest influence near the ends of words.

Parallel distributed processing has proven a powerful metaphor for speech perception and even contributed to the development of parallel (or neural-net) computers, which hold great promise for modeling human speech perception.

It has been shown that listeners can identify words just as soon as they have heard enough of the acoustic signal to eliminate other potential candidates. The fact that recognition can occurr before the end of the word has been presented is powerful evidence of the important contribution of top-down processing in speech perception.

For Further Reading

Elman, J., & McClelland, J. (1984). Speech perception as a cognitive process: The interactive activation model. In N. Lass (Ed.), *Speech and Language: Advances in Basic Research and Practice* (Vol. 10). New York: Academic Press.

McClelland, J., Rumelhart, D., and the PDP Research Group. (1986). *Parallel Distributed Processing: Explorations in the Microstructure of Cognition Volume 2: Psychological and Biological Models.* Cambridge, MA: MIT Press.

Rumelhart, D., McClelland, J., and the PDP Research Group. (1986). *Parallel Distributed Processing: Explorations in the Microstructure of Cognition Volume 1: Foundations.* Cambridge, MA: MIT Press.

REVIEW QUESTIONS

1. Briefly explain the difference between top-down versus bottom-up methods of perceptual processing.

2. Is identifying whether a particular sound sequence represents a word or not in a particular language an example of bottom-up or top-down processing?

3. What would be some of the advantages of being able to speak to a computer, rather than having to communicate via a keyboard?

4. What is the main difference between parallel and serial processing?

5. While the computer has been used extensively as a metaphor for the human brain over the last several decades, how have things changed recently?

CHAPTER

11

Studies of Infant Speech Perception

LEARNING OBJECTIVES

While we usually consider that children have to learn both to produce and perceive speech, in this chapter some of the evidence for innate speech processing in infants is presented. Speech perception seems to be a combination of both "nature" and "nurture," since some sound contrasts for which there is an innate perceptual basis undergo change with increasing exposure to a particular language. Some new sound contrasts may be acquired, and other sound constrasts may even be lost in the adult speaker. These concepts are the basis for exploring the development process in the following chapter.

Innate Versus Learned

One of the areas of speech perception that has undergone the most development in the past two decades is concerned with how very young children treat speech and nonspeech sounds. Popular understanding holds that speech is learned like any other motor behavior is, such as walking—that is, through a process of successful attempts that are rewarded and errors that are punished. But infant speech studies have shown that, at least for perception, the child does not come into the world a tabular rasa (blank slate)—there is a great deal of evidence that human infants are born with the capacity for categorizing many speech sounds in specialized ways. In other words, at birth children can already perform many of the rudimentary processes involved in speech perception. There seems to be a genetic underpinning for speech perception.

While this may be surprising at first, it is also surprising to learn that very young infants also naturally produce a walking-like response when stimulated lightly on the foot—a so-called stepping reflex. This response soon disappears and only reappears at a later point when the child actually begins to walk. In other words, there also seems to be some genetic organization for the rudiments of walking, which popular understanding also holds to be entirely learned.

A great deal of research has investigated speech perception in young infants. It is beyond the scope of the present chapter to provide a complete overview of this research. Rather, we will concentrate on some of the major findings and leave it up to the interested reader to delve into some of the fascinating studies in this area.

To summarize the present state of knowledge in this broad field of research: the infant seems to be born with certain general capacities for organizing many of the sounds of speech that are used in the world's various languages. It seems as if *all children everywhere* have the same perceptual capacities at birth. (And perhaps there is no greater evidence from science for the absurdity of linguistic strife.) Over the first year of life these perceptual capacities are modified by exposure to a particular language (or languages, as the case may be).

Yet, researchers have also demonstrated that infants of only a few weeks prefer to listen to their parental language, rather than some foreign language. Thus infants already demonstrate some influence of their native language from birth, possibly because of some exposure to speech sounds while still in the womb.

An important concept to understand in studying infant speech perception is the notion that a language can employ many different types of sound distinctions. The capacity to distinguish certain speech sounds may be present at birth, or speech perception may have to undergo a certain amount of change before it is adjusted to a distinction as it is used in a particular language. Other types of sound distinctions seem to be entirely learned, and there seems to be no innate support for these types of distinctions. In other words, there are roughly three types of sounds used in the world's languages: (a) sounds for which there is already a certain innate capacity to distinguish; (b) sounds which vary on a dimension for which there is some innate capacity, but which require some fine-tuning through experience; and (c) sounds for which there does not appear to be innate perceptual underpinnings.

Having provided a general conceptual framework, let us consider just two experiments in infant speech perception in order to gain a better idea about the scientific evidence for the statements made above.

Experimental Evidence

The first experiment that we'll discuss was actually one of the pioneering studies in this area. In the early 1970s Peter Eimas and his colleagues conducted a speech perception experiment with young infants from 1 to 4 months old (Eimas, Siqueland, Jusczyk, & Vigorito, 1971). These researchers employed three different sets of speech sounds (/pa/ and /ba/) that varied along the dimension of voice onset time (which you will recall from previous chapters). One pair of sounds had VOTs of 20 and 40 ms (milliseconds). As discussed in Chapter 5 on Categorical Perception, about 30 ms of VOT is the point at which voiced sounds change into voiceless sounds, and vice versa. Speech stimuli with a VOT of 20 ms (which is less than 30 ms) sounded like *bah*, while the stimuli with a VOT of 40 ms (which is more than 30 ms) sounded like *pah*. In another pair, the VOTs were 0 and 20 ms; in other words both stimuli sounded like *bah*.

In the third pair the VOTs were 60 and 80 ms, so both stimuli sounded like *pah*.

You are probably wondering how infants "told" the experimenters what they heard in a perceptual experiment, since they cannot yet speak. The researchers in this study used an ingenious method called *nonnutritive sucking* to investigate the infants' perception. As you already know, infants naturally like to suck on a pacifier, even though there is no bottle supplying nutrition. These researchers found they could measure this sucking response by outfitting a similar latex nipple with a pressure transducer that automatically records the number of times an infant sucks per some unit of time. Infants normally suck about 20 to 40 times per minute.

During the actual experiment, each time the apparatus recorded an instance of sucking, one sound of the stimulus pair was played. The infant discovers this interesting contingency. When infants hear something new in response to their sucking, they typically suck at a faster rate. The faster rate of sucking continues for several minutes and then returns to the baseline rate, as the child becomes familiar or habituated with the sound. Then a new sound is introduced and the experimenters look for an increase in the infants' sucking rate. In this manner, scientists can test what sounds are heard as "different" to the infant, because they will produce a faster sucking rate for these sounds.

The infants in Eimas and colleagues' study revealed faster sucking rates when the stimuli presented was changed from 20 to 40 ms VOT. In other words, the infants appeared to "perceive" the difference between /ba/ and /pa/ just like adult speakers do. But they did not produce faster sucking rates when the stimuli was changed from 0 to 20 ms VOT; nor from 60 to 80 ms VOT, even though both of these stimuli pairs vary by the same amount of 20 ms. Infants reacted to these stimuli just like adult speakers do; stimuli on the same side of the VOT continuum are heard as the same. In other words, Eimas and colleagues demonstrated the same *categorical perception* for the VOT dimension in infants that was previously discussed for adults (in the Chapter 5 on Categorical Perception).

As Eimas and his colleagues argued, it would be difficult to explain how an infant only 1 to 4 months after birth could have already learned to categorize speech sounds in an adult manner. In Eimas' opinion: "A simpler view is that categorization occurs because a child is born with perceptual mechanisms that are tuned to the properties of speech" (Eimas, 1974, p. 49). Similar experiments have since been conducted with infants even younger than 1 month, with similar results (e.g., Bertoncini, Bijelijas-Babic, Jusczyk, Kennedy, & Mehler, 1988).

While it may be surprising enough to learn that young infants can already discriminate between certain speech sounds in an adult manner, it is even more astounding to learn that in some instances, infants can discriminate speech sounds that adults cannot! Yet a number of experiments have demonstrated this to be the case for several different speech contrasts. For example, English-speaking adult listeners do not hear the difference between sounds such as *bah* which are produced with a negative VOT of 20 ms and a positive VOT of 60 ms, even though these two sounds are different phonemes in the Thai language. (In fact these two sounds may be the only difference between two different words in Thai—in other words they can form *minimal pairs*). Even though adult speakers of English do not discriminate these two sounds, Aslin, Pisoni, Hennesy, and Perey (1981) have shown that infants of English-speaking parents do. This suggests that not only does learning a language involve acquiring the ability to distinguish new sound contrasts, apparently it also involves a change in the ability to discriminate old ones.

Although we have only discussed infant perception research involving the VOT dimension thus far, there is additional research involving other speech contrasts such as the difference in place-of-articulation (Eimas, 1974). As was mentioned above, the change from infantlike speech categorization (which seems to be universal) to more adultlike perception (which is determined by a particular language) seems to begin during the first year of life (Strange, 1986; Werker & Tess, 1984).

Vowel Normalization in Infants

Above, we discussed an experiment that demonstrated the manner in which young infants can discriminate certain consonant sounds. Now we will consider an experiment that reveals infants' ability to perceive vowel sounds as similar. Speech perception not only involves the ability to discriminate between different speech sounds, but also the ability to ignore acoustic differences between linguistically similar sounds. In other words, not only do we have to hear the relevant differences in speech,we also have to ignore the irrelevant differences.

Kuhl (1979) has demonstrated that infants can react to the same vowel produced by different speakers as similar, despite the fact that the actual acoustic structure of vowels produced by different speakers can vary considerably. You will recall from Chapter 3 on vowel perception that this ability to compensate for differences due to different speakers of the same vowel is referred to as *vowel normalization.*

Kuhl employed a quite different experimental paradigm from that used by Eimas and his colleagues, since the infants she tested were somewhat older in age at 5 to 6 months. In this experimental paradigm, infants sit on their mother's laps where they feel secure. An experimenter holds the infants' attention with a toy. Repeating speech sounds such as *e e e* are presented over a loudspeaker. Then a change is introduced, such as changing the vowel to *ah*. When a sound change is presented, an electronic toy to the side is lit up and activated. Infants like this toy very much because it seems to be alive, since it moves all by itself. The children learn during a conditioning phase of the experiment that the toy will light up and move each time a sound change is presented over the loudspeaker. Eventually the infants learn to turn their head to look at the toy at their side each time a sound change is presented, even before the toy is activated. In this manner, another experimenter who is observing the child via a video monitor can investigate which sound contrasts the child hears as different.

Figure 11–1 presents two photographs of this head-turning method. In the top photograph an infant can be seen sitting on a mother's lap. To the left Dr. Kuhl is holding the infant's attention with a toy. Both the experimenter and the mother are wearing headphones so that they do not hear when the sound change occurs. This precaution is taken so that they don't influence the child's behavior. In the bottom photograph, note that, since a sound change has occurred, the infant has turned toward the visually reinforcing toy, which is lit up and now visible to the right of the picture.

Using this procedure Kuhl demonstrated that infants could correctly discriminate between different vowels (as demonstrated by the turns of their head to view the visual reinforcer before it was activated), and also did not react to differences between

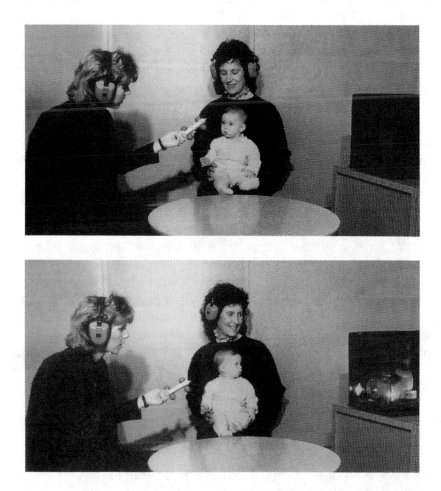

Figure 11–1. Head-turning procedure. Infants learn to turn their head to look at a toy on the right that lights up when a change in sound is detected. For the trial to be counted, the infant must turn his/her head *before* the toy lights up. In the top photograph, the infant, seated on his mother's lap. is distracted by Dr. Kuhl with a toy on the left. In the bottom photograph, a sound change has occurred and the infant has turned his head anticipating the toy which is now lit. (Reprinted with permission from Kuhl [1968]. Theoretical Contributions of Tests on Animals to the Special-Mechanisms Debate in Speech. *Experimental Biology, 45*, 233–265. Copyright 1986 by Springer-Verlag.)

the same vowel as produced by different speakers (i.e., no head turns). That is, the infants treated the vowel /i/ ("e e e") as the same whether they were produced by an adult male, adult female, or a child's voice.

Just two experiments that have investigated speech perception in the infant have been discussed here. There is actually a great deal of research in this area. Recently, investigators have also begun to focus more attention on the exact nature of the change from infantlike to adultlike speech perception. In the past, such research was limited by a lack of appropriate experimental methodologies for children who are no longer infants, but are not old enough to react just like adults. Some of this problem has been overcome to some extent, but many issues remain to be explored in this area. While there is a considerable body of research with 3- to 4-year-olds, the picture is still much less complete for 1- to 3-year-olds.

We have seen that humans are so adept at perceiving speech because we already come into the world at least partially equipped for this task. Hopefully, we can draw a lesson from the fact that all babies the world over seem to possess the same innate perceptual endowment. This fact should help us to emphasize the similarity between different peoples of the world and help us to minimize the differences resulting from different languages, religions, and cultures! Despite these differences that occur later in life, we all seem to come into the world with very similar brains.

Summary

We have seen how young children are capable of making certain sound distinctions necessary for speech perception from a very young age. They are also capable of recognizing the same vowel despite considerable acoustic differences due to different speakers' vocal tracts. This suggests that human infants already come into the world prepared to make many of the essential sound distinctions required for speech perception. Such innate perceptual capacities differ dramatically from the traditional and popular conception of speech perception that is only acquired slowly over time, in a similar manner to the mastery of speech production.

For Further Reading

Bertoncini, J., Bijeljas-Babic, R., Jusczyk, P., Kennedy, L., & Mehler, J. (1988). An investigation of young infants' perceptual representations of speech sounds. *Journal of Experimental Psychology: General, 117,* 21–33.

Eimas, P., & Miller, J. (1992). Organization in the perception of speech by young infants. *Psychological Science, 3*(6), 340–345.

Eimas, P., Siqueland, E., Jusczyk, P., & Vigorito, J. (1971). Speech perception in infants. *Science, 171,* 303–306.

Kuhl, P. (1979). The perception of speech in early infancy. In N. J. Lass (Ed.), *Speech and Language: Advances in Basic Research and Practice* (Vol. X). New York: Academic Press.

Kuhl, P. (1983). Perception of auditory equivalence classes for speech in early infancy. *Infant Behavior and Development, 6,* 263–285.

Kuhl, P. (1987). Perception of speech and sound in early infancy. In P. Salapatek & L. Cohen (Eds.), *Handbook of Infant Perception* (Vol. 2). New York: Academic Press.

Mehler, J. (1985). Language-related dispositions in early infancy. In J. Mehler & R. Fox (Eds.), *Neonate Cognition: Beyond the Blooming Buzzing Confusion.* Hillsdale, NJ: Erlbaum.

REVIEW QUESTIONS

1. Explain how a baby born in Newark, New Jersey can be shown to distinguish two different phonemes of Thai which that infant's parents hear as the same.

2. Does this chapter change the way you view speech perception? In what manner?

3. Does a young child hear the difference between an /i/ vowel spoken by a six-feet tall adult male and this same vowel spoken by its five-feet-two mother?

(continued)

(continued)

4. In Dr. Kuhl's head-turning experiment, why is it important that only trials, in which the infant turns its head **before** the toy has been activated, be counted?

5. Why do you think it is that some people refuse to believe that infants can perceive differences in sounds which their parents cannot? What is it that they seem to find disturbing?

CHAPTER

12

Development of
Speech Perception

LEARNING OBJECTIVES

The objective of this chapter is to explain how speech perception changes over the course of development. In the previous chapter we explored the universal innate speech processing capacities of the young infant. In the present
chapter we explore how speech perception makes this transition from young infant to adultlike. Recent evidence indicates that while this process is gradual, significant pro-gress
toward adultlike speech perception has already occurred by
1 year of age.

The change in speech perception at the other end of the
age spectrum is also briefly considered. Although increased
difficulty perceiving speech may be a symptom of advancing age, the precise manner is which speech is distorted
remains to be determined.

Phonetic to Phonemic
Speech Perception

In Chapter 11 we considered the universal speech perception capacities with which we are born. In this chapter we will discuss how these capacities develop with exposure to a particular language. We shall also briefly consider how speech perception abilities could potentially be affected by normal aging.

As was alluded to in the previous chapter, there were certain methodological issues that somewhat hampered research with younger children who are no longer infants. It is difficult to hold the attention of a child who is no longer content to sit quietly on mother's lap listening to speech sounds over a loudspeaker. Also, children younger than 3 years cannot yet be expected to provide reliable information about which speech sounds they heard. Thus it is difficult to test their ability to *identify* speech sounds, even though they can be tested for their *discrimination* (the ability to hear a difference between two sounds—see Chapter 5 on Categorical Perception).

Werker and colleagues have referred to this difference between the universal capacities that seem to be innate as the *phonetic* mode of perception, whereas *phonemic* perception refers to perception that is language-specific (Werker & Tess, 1984). These researchers have documented the disintegration of the ability to make speech contrasts from the Salish (an American Indian language) and Hindi languages, in children from English-speaking backgrounds, as a function of age. English-speaking children are born with the capacity to discriminate certain consonantal contrasts from these two languages. Thus at 6–8 months, English-speaking infants can distinguish place-of-articulation contrasts that are no longer distinguished by English-speaking adults.

As shown in Figure 12–1 from Werker and Tess (1984) this ability disintegrates progressively over the first year of age. However, children from Hindi or Salish backgrounds retain the ability to perceive these linguistic contrasts native to their language.

Werker and her colleagues have shown further that this effect of language input on perceptual abilities between about 6 and 12 months of age is not completely irreversible. That is, with enough training or with enough experience learning a second

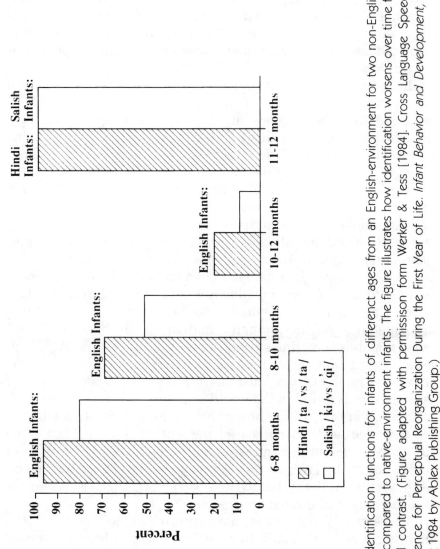

Figure 12–1. Identification functions for infants of differenct ages from an English-environment for two non-English sound contrasts compared to native-environment infants. The figure illustrates how identification worsens over time for nonnative sound contrast. (Figure adapted with permissison form Werker & Tess [1984]. *Cross Language Speech Perception: Evidence for Perceptual Reorganization During the First Year of Life. Infant Behavior and Development, 7,* 49–63. Copyright 1984 by Ablex Publishing Group.)

language, there is still some discrimination of difficult nonnative contrasts (Werker, 1989). (Good news for those of us who have spent years trying to learn another language!) Werker suggests that this developmental change between infancy and adulthood should be looked at as a "language-based reorganization" of phonemes rather than "an absolute loss of auditory sensitivity" (p. 58).

Evidence suggests that children begin to perceive speech in a native manner around their first year. Strange (1986) has pointed out that this is the same age at which children begin to produce their first words. While this *phonemic* speech perception begins around the first year of life, Strange (1986) suggests that children only perform truly adultlike identification by 4 years of age.

Werker and Polka (1993) have reviewed the work in this area and describe what they feel to be the consensus view of the developmental change in speech perception in terms of three stages. First, infants already come into the world with certain perceptual capacities for phonetic distinctions used in the world's languages. Infants have been shown capable of perceptual distinctions for sounds that are not used in their native language. (It is somewhat premature to state whether or not infants are capable of *all* the phonetic distinctions of the world's languages, as has sometimes been done in the literature. Although a significant number of contrasts have been investigated, this inventory does not yet adequately reflect the wide variety of speech sounds found in the world's languages.) Second, research with adult speakers has shown that "experience with a particular language leads to decreased perceptibility of at least some nonnative phonetic contrasts, and enhanced perception of native contrasts" (Werker & Polka, 1993, p. 83). Third, by the end of the first year, the influence of a particular language is seen on the perception of nonnative speech.

Polka and Werker (1994) have directed some research at the precise course of this shift in speech perception from universal/phonetic to language-specific/phonemic in the young child. Potentially such results on the shift to native-like speech perception are of concern to speech pathology since this shift presumably occurs during the stage at which a child might also develop of a link between internal speech sounds and graphemic symbols to be used in reading. However, we know precious little about the potential interaction of speech perception on reading skills. Let us simply point out here that such a link could and probably does occur. This area of investigation is important to audiology because it may help understand how speech perception differs in children whose limited hearing has impeded this change to nativelike speech perception. (See Chapter 14 on Disorders Affecting Speech Perception.)

Strange (1986) has summarized the basic facts about the development of speech perception as follows:

> Prelinguistic infants appear to have the capacity to discriminate all or most of the acoustic parameters of speech that differentiate the phonemes of the languages of the world. They perceive speech in terms of language-universal phonetic categories. By the end of the first year of life, as the child begins to use speech productively to convey meaning, speech perceptual patterns have already been constrained to some extent by the specific phonological structure of the native language. Native language contrasts continue to be perceptually differentiated (although there may be some collapsing of adult phonemic categories) while non-native contrast are no longer discriminated easily. Phonological processes in normal children continue to be refined throughout the early preschool years with perceptual differentiation of native contrasts usually preceding articulatory differentiation. By the time the child is four to five years old, adult-like language specific perceptual patterns appear to be well learned and perhaps automatic, although there are questions remaining about the malleability of such processes in the preadolescent years and beyond. (p. 23)

Normal Aging of Speech Perception

The important issue remains how speech perception might be affected by the normal aging process. Loss of hearing resulting from the normal process of aging is known as *presbycusis.* Difficulty understanding speech is a major complaint of older persons experiencing hearing loss. We will discuss how speech perception is affected by aphasia in Chapter 14 on Disorders Affecting Speech Perception.

It is not known precisely how speech perception is affected by aging. Evidence suggests that, similar to hearing loss patterns earlier in life, certain speech sounds are more vulnerable to hearing loss with age than others. Fricative sounds, which are somewhat weaker in amplitude, are more likely to be misperceived than vowel sounds, which are inherently louder. Certain sound contrasts, such as voiced versus voiceless and place-of-articulation, also appear more susceptible than others. But we are not yet capable of modeling hearing loss accurately.

There is some evidence in the literature that speech production is affected by age. Certainly, in a theory which posits a link between motor speech production and speech perception, we might also expect speech perception to change with age despite intact hearing.

Summary

Speech perception changes from a universal mode at birth to one which has already adapted to the particular native language by the first year of life. The universal speech processing ability present at birth is often referred to as the *phonetic mode* of perception, whereas the *phonemic mode* of perception refers to speech processing that has adapted to a particular language. Ongoing research is attempting to more accurately chart the timetable and determine the precise nature of this important change in speech perception.

For Further Reading

Goodman, J., & Nusbaum, H. (1993). *The transition from speech sounds to spoken words: The development of speech perception.* Cambridge, MA: MIT Press.

Jusczyk, P. (1985). On characterizing the development of speech perception. In J. Mehler & R. Fox (Eds.), *Neonate cognition: Beyond the blooming, buzzing confusion.* Hillsdale, NJ: Erlbaum.

Kuhl, P., Williams, K., Lacerda, F., Stevens, K., & Lindblom, B. (1992). Linguistic experience alters phonetic perception in infants by 6 months of age. *Science, 255,* 1003–1010.

Polka, L., & Werker, J. (1994). Developmental changes in the perception of non-native vowel contrasts. *Journal of Experimental Psychology: Human Perception and Performance, 20,* 421–435.

Strange, W. (1986). Speech input and the development of speech perception. In J. Kavanaugh (Ed.). *Otitis Media and Child Development.* Parkton, MD: York Press.

Werker, J. (1986). The effect of multilingualism on phonetic perceptual flexibility. *Applied Psychophysics, 7,* 141–156.

Werker, J. (1989). Becoming a native listener. *American Scientist, 77,* 54–59.

Werker, J., & Pegg, J. (1992). Infant speech perception and phonological acquisition. In C. Ferguson, L. Menn, & C. Stoel-Gammon (Eds.), *Phonological Development: Models, Research and Implications.* Parkton, MD: York Press.

Werker, J., & Polka, L. (1993). Developmental changes in speech perception: New challenges and new directions. *Journal of Phonetics, 21,* 83–101.

Werker, J., & Tess, R. (1984). Cross-language speech perception: Evidence for perceptual reorganization during the first year of life. *Infant Behavior and Development, 7,* 49–63.

REVIEW QUESTIONS

1. Explain the difference between the phonemic and the phonetic modes of speech perception.

2. Which of the two (i.e., phonetic or phonemic) refers to the speech perception of young infants?

3. How is perception different in very young infants compared to adults?

4. Why do you think speech perception changes as infants develop and get older? In other words, why couldn't infants just come into the world already prepared to perceive the phonemes of their native language?

5. What are the speech sounds that seem to be more vulnerable to hearing loss?

CHAPTER

13

Speech Perception in Animals

LEARNING OBJECTIVES

This chapter is devoted to consideration of the speech processing capacities of animals. By comparing the nature of speech processing in animals to that of humans, we stand to gain better insight into how humans have become especially adapted for the use of speech. Some research has uncovered remarkable similarities in the discrimination functions of chinchillas for certain speech contrasts to those for human listeners. This suggests that human speech perception has a basis in some sound distinctions general to the mammalian species.

Animals and Human Speech

Surely at one time or another you've heard the claim: "My pet understands me when I talk to him." Perhaps you've even made a similar claim yourself. In this chapter we will briefly consider speech processing in animals. While we won't provide an exact answer to what degree animals process human speech, many mammals do indeed seem to possess some basic abilities for processing speech.

Should we feel threatened that other animals demonstrate some rudimentary underpinnings for human speech perception? No, rather than considering animals more human when we consider this research, perhaps we should remember that we are also one form of mammal—albeit highly evolved and intelligent. Human speech probably employs sound distinctions based on basic perceptual capacities general to all mammals.

It should really come as no surprise that mammals can process some rudimentary sound distinctions basic to human speech. Yet, some people felt threatened by the idea that other animals might perceive some aspects of human speech. Apparently they feel they are less human, or somewhat less divine, when other animals are deemed capable of some processing of human language. The fact that our simian cousins seem to comprehend human speech is sometimes offered as evidence of human's evolution.

As interesting and as stimulating as such a discussion might be, this controversy will not be treated further. Rather, we will turn our attention to some of the experimental evidence which supports the notion of speech perception capacities in animals. The discussion will largely be limited to the perceptual capacities of one animal species (the chinchilla) on one acoustic dimension of human speech (the voicing dimension).

Experimental Evidence from Chinchillas

In one experiment chinchillas were trained to respond differently to naturally spoken occurrences of /t/ and /d/. They were taught to avoid a mild shock by moving across their cage to the other half of the grill floor. Reward for correct performance consisted of "free" drinking water. Training on natural speech stimuli was even found to generalize to new stimuli produced by different speakers.

In a second experiment synthetic stimuli were presented in an *identification* task (Kuhl & Miller, 1978). It was found that the phonetic VOT boundary between /t/ and /d/ was very similar for chinchillas and for adult speakers of English——both were approximately 35 ms. (The boundary is operationally defined as the point where identification responses are evenly divided between the two choices. See Chapter 5 on Categorical Perception.) This VOT boundary value for alveolars is also in good agreement with previous results from Lisker and Abramson (1970).

These results essentially demonstrate categorical perception in chinchillas. The results are somewhat surprising in that *categorical perception* was previously thought to be one of the hallmarks of uniquely human speech processing. While the perception for the sounds of speech may indeed still be special or quite different than that for other sounds, it can no longer be argued to be uniquely human.

Kuhl and Miller (1978) interpret their results in the following manner: "The fact that the chinchillas respond to the synthetic speech as though an abrupt qualitative change occurs in the short voicing-lag region of the VOT continuum at precisely the place where many languages separate two phonemic categories lends support to the idea that speech-sound oppositions were selected to be highly distinctive to the auditory system" (p. 72).

In other words, languages of the world have probably taken advantage of sound differences that are naturally discriminated by mammals. Since speech perception is a complicated process, it is better to exploit every available naturally occurring advantage.

Kuhl (1981) has also obtained *discrimination* data for the chinchilla on the same /da/-/ta/ continuum using an "up-down threshold tracking procedure." The data from this experiment revealed that the chinchillas were most sensitive to a change in the stimuli at 30 ms VOT. Like human listeners, the chinchillas' discrimination abilities were similar to their identification abilities. (We have previously discussed discrimination versus identification.) Chinchillas reacted similarly to human listeners in both discrimination and identification.

Other Animal Species

Speech discrimination abilities have also been demonstrated for other animal species (e.g., in dogs—Baru, 1975; in monkeys—Sinott, Beecher, Moody & Stebbins, 1976; Waters & Wilson,

1976). Of course, some birds such as parrots and mynahs are also capable of imitating human speech. Klatt and Stefanski (1974) have investigated production of speech in the mynah. This ability to produce understandable speech in turn implies that these birds are able to extract from human speech the basic sound elements to be imitated.

Future experimentation is necessary to delineate the similarities and differences between human and animal perception of speech. Very similar results have been obtained with both humans and chinchillas for the VOT dimension. Such results may ultimately relate to basic temporal resolution properties of the mammalian nervous system. It is still quite possible that human and animal listeners will perform very differently on a different acoustic dimension of speech such as the one relating to place-of-articulation.

In any case, animal studies help to place speech perception within the context of human evolution. Such studies may eventually help gain a much better understanding of human perception through comparison with animals. Data from such experiments will help us to characterize what is uniquely human in the process of speech perception.

Although some students might object to the laboratory conditions to which animals must be subjected in order to obtain relevant data, the important scientific value of such experiments should not be underestimated. While chinchillas have demonstrated a rather uncanny ability to perceive human speech, they still are probably not likely to be signing informed subject consent forms any time soon!

Summary

Human speech seems to have taken advantage of certain sound distinction properties that are general to the mammalian species. This is not to imply that all mammals are capable of all sound distinctions required for speech. It suggests, rather, that speech exploits basic acoustic distinctions, which may ultimately relate to the physiologically based limitations of the mammalian nervous system. It also helps to remind us that while we typically think of speech an exclusively human, we share some of our sound processing capabilities with other species. Whereas we may be the only animal talking, we are apparently not the only animal listening!

For Further Reading

Baru, A.V. (1975). Discrimination of synthesized vowels /a/ and /I/ with varying parameters in dog. In G. Fant and M.A. Tatham (Eds.), *Auditory Analysis and the Perception of Speech*. London: Academic Press.

Klatt, D., & Stefanski, R., (1974). How does a mynah bird imitate human speech? *Journal of the Acoustical Society of America, 55*, 822–832.

Kuhl, P. (1981). Discrimination of speech by nonhuman animals: Basic auditory sensitivities conducive to the perception of speech-sound categories. *Journal of the Acoustical Society of America, 70*, 340–349.

Kuhl, P., & Miller, J. (1975). Speech perception by the chinchilla: Voiced-voiceless distinction in alveolar plosive consonants. *Science, 190*, 69–72.

Kuhl, P., & Miller, J. (1978). Speech perception by the chinchilla: Identification functions for synthetic VOT stimuli. *Journal of the Acoustical Society of America, 63*, 905–917.

Sinott, J., Beecher, M., Moody, D., & Stebbins, W. (1976). Speech sound discrimination by monkeys and humans. *Journal of the Acoustical Society of America, 60*, 687–695.

Waters, R., & Wilson, W.A. Jr. (1976). Speech perception by rhesus monkeys: The voicing distinction in synthesized labial and velar stop consonants. *Perception and Psychophysics, 19*, 285- 289.

REVIEW QUESTIONS

1. What is surprising about the fact that chinchilla can be trained to discriminate sounds on two sides of a 35-ms VOT boundary?

2. Does this discovery mean that chinchillas will soon be hired as radio announcers? Why not? (In other words, what are they still lacking?)

3. While discrimination results for chinchillas are similar for the VOT dimension, this chapter suggests that they

(continued)

(continued)

may be very different for some other speech sound contrast. What is the speech sound contrast referred to in the chapter? What are the reasons this particular sound contrast might produce very different results for the chinchilla?

4. What kinds of evidence do people typically use to support the claim that their pet "understands" human speech? What do you think about this evidence from a scientific perspective?

CHAPTER

14

Disorders Affecting Speech Perception

LEARNING OBJECTIVES

This chapter considers three different speech disorders which are also known to affect speech perception: adult aphasia, hearing impairment, and specific linguistic impairments. The purpose of the chapter is to begin to familiarize the reader with the speech perception difficulties that often accompany various speech and language disorders.

In this last chapter we will consider a few speech disorders that affect speech perception. These disorders are: adult aphasia, hearing impairment, and specific language impairment. These are only a few representative speech-language pathologies that also affect speech perception. Because of the close link between production and perception, the two are often jointly perturbed. The degree to which they are independent systems remains to be clearly determined.

The three disorders that have been chosen for more detailed consideration here are merely chosen to sensitize the reader to some of the ways in which speech perception can be perturbed. While much important information is still lacking in this area, we can begin to put together some of the pieces of the puzzle.

Adult Aphasia

Aphasia is a language disorder that results from some form of insult to the brain. Because aphasia has somewhat different effects when it occurs in adult speakers who have already mastered their native language than in children who are still in the process of language acquisition, it is necessary to distinguish between adult and childhood aphasia.

In adult speakers, aphasia also typically has different symptoms according to whether the anterior or posterior portion of the left hemisphere is damaged. The traditional neurological landmark that distinguishes anterior from posterior is the Rolandic fissure. *Broca's aphasia* may result from anterior damage in the left hemisphere, while *Wernicke's aphasia* can result from damage to the posterior portion. Wernicke's aphasics are generally thought to experience more difficulty in the linguistic organization of phonemes, but are typically still fluent speakers who do not appear to have difficulty with the motor organization of speech. Yet, they often reveal difficulties in comprehending speech and language. Broca's aphasics, in contrast, typically experience difficulty in the motor production of speech despite apparently intact phonemic organization and good comprehension. Broca's aphasics often repeat and correct themselves, which seems to reveal that they are typically aware of their speech problem.

Given these general tendencies, one might expect Wernicke's aphasics to experience greater difficulties in perceiving speech, since they generally seem to have more difficulty understanding spoken language. Carl Wernicke (1874, 1908) expressed this in the following manner: "In spoken words he hears either a confused noise that has no meaning for him or, at best, a language completely foreign to him."

A number of investigations have compared phonemic perception in Broca's and Wernicke's aphasics and failed to find the clear cut difference between these two types of aphasia in a manner consistent with theoretical claims (Basso, Casati, & Vignolo, 1977; Blumstein, Goodglass, & Baker, 1977; Keller, Rothenberger, & Goepfert, 1982; Ryalls, 1987a.) Such results suggest that either speech production and speech perception are inextricably linked at all stages of cognitive elaboration (as claimed by Brown, 1977); or that theory has not yet accurately characterized differences between these two main types of aphasia. It is clear, however, that further studies of speech perception in this disorder could shed more light on the nature of aphasia.

Hearing Impairment

We all have some notion of how hearing impairment affects normal speech production, either through personal association or through the media. The degree that speech is perturbed varies somewhat according to the degree of hearing loss. But of equal, if not greater, importance is whether the loss occurred before or after the individual had acquired language. The terms that refer to this difference are *pre-lingual* and *post-lingual* respectively.

Usually, the word *deaf* is avoided these days, since this term implies absolutely no hearing whatsoever, which is actually rare. But it is also true that some persons with profound hearing loss who have vigorously adopted sign language may actually prefer to describe themselves as members of the "deaf community" even though they may have some residual hearing. They tend to view "deafness" culturally, rather than in terms of the associated disability.

Although there is quite a bit of research literature on speech production in individuals with hearing impairment (see Osberger & McGarr [1982] for an excellent overview), there is only rudimentary information on the exact manner in which hearing impairment affects speech perception (Dubno, Dirks, & Langhofer, 1982; Owens, Talbott, & Schubert, 1968). While some effects are predictable, such as the fact that inherently louder sounds such as vowels are easier to distinguish than inherently softer sounds such as fricatives, other effects are not. For example, it is often pointed out that the fundamental frequency of speech is typically the lowest frequency of speech. Lower frequencies tend to be relatively less affected by hearing loss—which usually takes a greater toll in the higher frequencies. This might suggest that individuals with hearing impairment should produce relatively intact fundamental frequency contours. However, a higher-than-average fundamental frequency is one of the most frequent speech disturbances encountered in the speech of those with impaired hearing. This in turn suggests that not all speech production problems encountered in individuals with hearing impairment are a direct reflection of the perceptual disturbance. It has been suggested that abnormally high fundamental frequency in speakers with hearing impairment may result from greater vocal effort or a higher degree of psychological stress associated with speech production.

The development and rather widespread use of cochlear implants offers a new opportunity for investigating the development of speech perception with unparalleled precision. In some cases, children have basically no speech perception since speech was not accessible through hearing, and yet they are able to make dramatic improvements over a relatively short period of time. Research in this area could shed light on just how general auditory abilities are molded into the specialized perceptual processes required for rapid speech.

Specific Language Impairment

There are currently a number of terms being employed to describe various disorders in children that also affect speech perception. At present, it is not clear to what degree these clinical entities are distinct and to what degree they overlap. For example it is not clear exactly how speech perception problems, that are not a result of hearing impairment, referred to as *disorders of central processing* (Katz, Stecker, & Henderson, 1992), are distinct from the speech perception problems associated with the disorder referred to as *specific linguistic impairment.* While one would not expect other associated language problems in those with disorders of central processing sometimes such persons have undergone little formal language testing.

Since a lot of confusion seems to prevail in the use of these terms, as well as in the use of older terms like "dysphasic," "childhood aphasic," and so on, there is a need for formal clinical tests capable of distinguishing these syndromes.

The work of Dr. Paula Tallal has especially served to bring the speech perception problems of some young children who have difficulty acquiring language to the forefront. Tallal's work (reviewed in Tallal, Miller, & Fitch, 1993) suggests that the speech perception difficulties of some children with language delay, are due to a more general processing problem with stimuli that change rapidly in a brief period of time. The finding that at least some of these children not only require longer intervals to distinguish auditory stimuli, but also demonstrate a similar processing impairment in the visual mode, suggests that there is a common temporal denominator. Tallal and colleagues have provided an overview on timing as a critical factor (Tallal, Miller, & Fitch, 1993).

Since timing seems to be implicated, we can expect that speech-related events reflecting large spectral changes over a short unit of time (such as the place of articulation distinction in consonants) would be especially perceptually challenging for these children. Other longer term changes, such as the formant structure for vowel sounds, might be expected to be less difficult. Frumkin and Papin (1980) have found differences in subgroups of children with language impairment—one group had more difficulty with steady-state vowels, while the other group had more difficulty with the rapidly changing formant transitions for consonants. Yet, if timing is indeed a more critical factor, as suggested by Tallal and colleagues (1993), one might expect that steady-state vowels are less perceptually taxing than the rapidly changing formant transitions that signal consonants. Sussman (1993) has suggested that the perceptual problems of children with language impairments are more reflective of left hemisphere processing limitations than a lack of sensitivity to formant transitions per se.

In another vein, Leonard and colleagues (1992) investigated the potential association between morphological limitations of children with specific linguistic impairment and their perceptual processing of speech. They found that the children in their study had more difficulty in discriminating speech stimuli whose contrastive portions were longer than their noncontrasting portions. Such results suggest an even tighter link between grammar and acoustics than previously conceived.

Children with specific linguistic impairments are presently the focus of intense scrutiny. This research effort is likely to yield a much more detailed picture of the various clinical disorders clustered about these various speech and language disorders.

As suggested at the beginning of this chapter, there are a variety of speech-language disorders that perturb perceptual processing for speech. We have briefly discussed just three examples here. Since the tight link between speech production and speech perception has been a reccurring theme in this book, one might anticipate potential perceptual ramifications to accompany any disorder that affects normal production of articulate speech.

In summary, we have considered some of the basic perceptual processes involved in the normal rapid understanding of speech. Speech is typically understood as fast as it can be produced (and sometimes faster, when words are understood before their acoustic signal is completed). Speech can often be increased beyond normal production rates and still be understood by most listeners. Even though we touched on most of the important basic aspects of speech perception, this is an area of inquiry that is still developing rapidly. Yet there is not even a consensus on what constitutes the basic temporal unit of speech perception (Kent, 1992).

Digital technologies have allowed much simpler manipulations of speech signals, and there are now contemporary models of speech perception more representative of human neural processing in general. These two factors together, combined with our curiosity about ourselves and our language which makes us human, suggest that our understanding of human speech perception will continue to evolve in a vigorous manner well into the 21st century.

The reader who wants to keep abreast of these exciting developments will now have to make the step over into consulting the scientific journals. It is hoped that this book has prepared you to make this transition, and you are now a little more aware of just how complicated this everyday process of speech perception is, that we all take so for granted.

Summary

According to theoretical claims about aphasia, it is expected that Broca's aphasics should reveal essentially intact speech perception in contrast to Wernicke's aphasics. Yet, several studies have not revealed significantly different speech perception results between these two different clinical syndromes. This suggests that our present model of aphasia does not accurately portray speech perception.

The detrimental effect that hearing impairment has on speech perception does not seem to be completely based on acoustic principles. While fundamental frequency is usually produced in the lower frequencies, which are typically less affected by hearing loss than the higher frequencies, the speech of persons with hearing impairment often has an abnormally high fundamental frequency.

Tallal and colleagues have suggested that some children with speech and language problems require longer than normal timing differences to distinguish certain sound stimuli. This suggests that such children would have much less difficulty with the relatively slower changing formants that typify vowels than with the more rapidly changing acoustic information that specifies consonants. Yet, at least one study has identified children who have just as much trouble with the latter as with the former.

Experimental results considered in this chapter suggest that while we are beginning to gain an idea of how certain speech disorders also affect perception, we still have a long way to go.

For Further Reading

Adult Aphasia and Speech Perception

Blumstein, S., Goodglass, H., & Baker, E. (1977). Phonological factors in auditory comprehension in aphasia. *Neuropsychologia, 15*, 371–384.

Ryalls, J. (1987). Vowel perception in aphasia. *Clinical Linguistics & Phonetics, 1*(1), 91–95.

Hearing Impairment and Speech Perception

Dubno, J., Dirks, D., & Langhofer, L. (1982). Evaluation of hearing-impaired listeners using a nonsense syllable test. II. Syllable recognition and consonant confusion patterns. *Journal of Speech and Hearing Research, 25,* 141–148.

Osberger, M. J., & McGarr, N. (1982). Speech production characteristics of the hearing impaired. In N. Lass (Ed.), *Speech and Language: Advances in Basic Research and Practice* (Vol. 8, pp. 221–283), New York: Academic Press.

Owens, E., Talbott, C., & Schubert, E. (1968). Vowel discrimination of hearing-impaired listeners. *Journal of Speech and Hearing Research, 11,* 648–655.

Speech Perception in Children with Specific Language Impairment:

Frumkin, B., & Rapin, I. (1980). Perception of vowels and consonant-vowels of varying duration in language impaired children. *Neuropsychologia, 18,* 443–454.

Leonard, L., McGregor, K., & Allen, G. (1992). Grammatical morphology and speech perception in children with Specific Language Impairment. *Journal of Speech and Hearing Research, 35,* 1076–1085.

Sussman, J. (1993). Perception of formant transition cues to place of articulation in children with language impairments. *Journal of Speech and Hearing Research, 36,* 1286–1299.

Tallal, P., Miller, S., & Fitch, R. (1993). Neurobiological basis of speech: A case for the preeminence of temporal processing. In P. Tallal, A. Gallaburda, R. Llinas, & C. von Euler (Eds.), *Temporal Processing in the Nervous System* (pp. 27–47). *Annals of the New York Academy of Sciences, 682.*

REVIEW QUESTIONS

1. In which type of aphasia would we expect to see relatively intact speech perception?

2. Do studies bear out the expected difference between the speech perception of Broca's versus Wernicke's aphasics?

3. Why is it surprising that so many persons with hearing impairment speak with an abnormally high fundamental frequency?
4. Tallal and her colleagues have suggested that there is one overriding factor that accounts for the speech perception difficulties of children with language delay. What is this factor?
5. If this factor does account for such children's speech perception difficulties, would we expect them to have more difficulties with consonants or vowels? Why?

References

Aslin, R., Pisoni, D., Hennessy, B., & Perey, A. (1981). Discrimination of voice onset time by human infants: New findings and implications for the effect of early experience. *Child Development, 52,* 1135–1145.

Baru, A.V. (1975). Discrimination of synthesized vowels /a/ and /I/ with varying parameters in dog. In G. Fant and M.A. Tatham (Eds.), *Auditory Analysis and the Perception of Speech.* London: Academic Press.

Basso, A., Casati, G., & Vignolo, L. (1977). Phonemic identification defect in aphasia. *Cortex, 13,* 84–95.

Bertoncini, J., Bijeljas-Babic, R., Jusczyk, P., Kennedy, L., & Mehler, J. (1988). An investigation of young infants' perceptual representations of speech sounds. *Journal of Experimental Psychology: General, 117,* 21–33.

Blumstein, S. (1978). The perception of speech in pathology and ontogeny. In A. Caramazza & E. Zurif (Eds.), *Language Acquisition and Language Breakdown: Parallels and Divergencies.* Baltimore, MD: The Johns Hopkins University Press.

Blumstein, S. (1986). On acoustic invariance in speech. In J. Perkell & D. Klatt (Eds.), *Invariance and Variability in Speech Processes.* Hillsdale, NJ: Erlbaum.

Blumstein, S., & Cooper, W. (1974). Hemispheric processing of intonation. *Cortex, 10*, 146–158.

Blumstein, S., Goodglass, H., & Baker, E. (1977). Phonological factors in auditory comprehension in aphasia. *Neuropsychologia, 15*, 19–30.

Blumstein, S., Goodglass, H., & Tarter, V. (1975). The reliability of ear advantage in dichotic listening. *Brain and Language, 2*, 226–236.

Blumstein, S., Cooper, W., Goodglass, H., Statlender, S., & Gottlieb, J. (1980). Production deficits in aphasia: A voice-onset time analysis. *Brain and Language, 9*, 153–170.

Blumstein, S., & Stevens, K. (1979). Acoustic invariance in speech production: Evidence from measurements of the spectral characteristics of stop consonants. *Journal of the Acoustical Society of America, 66*(4), 1001–1017.

Blumstein, S., & Stevens, K. (1980). Perceptual invariance and onset spectra for stop consonants in different vowel environments. *Journal of the Acoustical Society of America, 67*(2), 648–662.

Borden, G., Harris, K., & Raphael, L. (1994). *Speech Science Primer: Physiology, Acoustics and Perception of Speech* (3rd Edition). Baltimore, MD: Williams & Wilkins.

Broadbent, D. (1954). The role of auditory localization in attention and memory span. *Journal of Experimental Psychology, 47*, 191–196.

Brown, J. (1977). *Mind, Brain, and Consciousness: The Neuropsychology of Cognition. Perspectives in Neurolinguistics, Neuropsychology, and Psycholinguistics Series.* New York: Academic Press.

Chomsky, N., & Halle, M. (1968). *The Sound Pattern of English.* New York: Harper & Row.

Cole, R., & Jakimik, J. (1978). Understanding speech: How words are heard. In G. Underwood (Ed.), *Strategies of Information Processing.* New York: Academic Press.

Cooper, W. (1974). Adaptation of phonetic feature analyzers for place of articulation. *Journal of the Acoustical Society of America, 56*, 617–627.

Cutting, J. (1972). Plucks and bows are categorically perceived, sometimes. *Perception and Psychophysics, 31*, 462–476.

Delgutte, B. (1980). Representation of speech-like sounds in the discharge patterns of auditory-nerve fibers. *Journal of the Acoustical Society of America, 68*(3), 843–857.

Divenyi, P., & Effron, R. (1979). Spectral versus temporal features in dichotic listening. *Brain and Language, 7*, 375–386.

Dubno, J., Dirks, D., & Langhofer, L. (1982). Evaluation of hearing-impaired listeners using a nonsense-syllable test. *Journal of Speech & Hearing Research, 25*, 141–148.

Eimas, P. (1974). Auditory and linguistic processing of cues for place of articulation by infants. *Perception and Psychophysics, 16*, 513–521.

Eimas, P., Cooper, W., & Corbit, J., (1973). Some properties of linguistic feature detectors. *Perception and Psychophysics, 13*, 247–252.

Eimas, P., & Corbit, J. (1973). Selective adaptation of linguistic feature detectors. *Perception and Psychophysics, 4*, 99–109.

Eimas, P., & Miller, J. (1978). Effects of selective adaptation on the perception of speech and visual forms: Evidence for feature detectors. In R. D. Walk & H. L. Pick Jr. (Eds.), *Perception and Experience.* New York: Plenum.

Eimas, P., & Miller, J. (1992). Organization in the perception of speech by young infants. *Psychological Science, 3*(6), 340–345.

Eimas, P., Siqueland, E., Jusczyk, P., & Vigorito, J. (1971). Speech perception in infants. *Science, 171*, 303–306.

Elman, J., & McClelland, J. (1984). Speech perception as a cognitive process: The interactive activation model. In N. Lass (Ed.), *Speech and Language: Advances in Basic Research and Practice* (Vol. 10). New York: Academic Press.

Fodor, J. (1983). *The Modularity of Mind.* Cambridge, MA: MIT Press.

Forrest, K., Weismer, G., Milenkovic, P., & Dougall, R. (1988). Statistical analysis of word-initial voiceless obstruents: Preliminary data. *Journal of the Acoustical Society of America, 84*(1), 115–123.

Fromkin, V. (1971). The non-anomalous nature of anomalous utterances. *Language, 47*, 27–52.

Fromkin, V. (Ed.). (1973). *Speech Errors as Linguistic Evidence.* The Hague, Netherlands: Mouton.

Frumkin, B., & Rapin, I. (1980). Perception of vowels and consonant-vowels of varying duration in language impaired children. *Neuropsychologia, 18*, 443–454.

Geffen, G., & Quinn, K. (1984). Hemispheric specialization and ear advantages in processing speech. *Psychological Bulletin, 96*(2), 273–291.

Goodman, J., & Nusbaum, H. (1993). *The transition from speech sounds to spoken words: The development of speech perception.* Cambridge, MA: MIT Press.

Haggard, M. (1971). Encoding and the REA for speech signals. *Quarterly Journal of Experimental Psychology, 23*, 34–45.

Jakobson, R., Fant, G., & Halle, M. (1963). *Preliminaries to Speech Analysis: The Distinctive Features and Their Correlates.* (Original work published 1952) Cambridge, MA: MIT Press.

Jusczyk, P. (1985). On characterizing the development of speech perception. In J. Mehler & R. Fox (Eds.), *Neonate Cognition: Beyond the Blooming, Buzzing Confusion.* Hillsdale, NJ: Erlbaum.

Katz, J., Stecker, N., & Henderson, D. (1992). *Central Auditory Precessing: A Transdisciplinary View.* St. Louis, MO: Mosby.

Keller, E., Rothenberger A., & Goepfert, M. (1982). Perceptual discrimination of vowels in aphasia. *Archiv für Psychiatrie und Nervenkrakenheiten, 231,* 339–357.

Kent, R. (1992). Auditory processing of speech. In J. Katz, N. Stecker, & D. Henderson (Eds.), *Central Auditory Processing: A Transdisciplinary View* (Chapter 8, pp. 93–106). St. Louis, MO: Mosby Year Book.

Kent, R., & Read, C. (1992). *The Acoustic Analysis of Speech.* San Diego, CA: Singular.

Kewley-Port, D. (1983). Time-varying features as correlates of place of articulation in stop consonants. *Journal of the Acoustical Society of America, 73,* 322–335.

Kimura, D. (1961). Cerebral dominance and the perception of verbal stimuli. *Canadian Journal of Psychology, 15,* 166–171.

Kimura, D. (1967). Functional asymmetry of the brain in dichotic listening. *Cortex, 3,* 163–168.

Klatt, D., & Stefanski, R., (1974). How does a mynah bird imitate human speech? *Journal of the Acoustical Society of America, 55,* 822–832.

Kuhl, P. (1979). The perception of speech in early infancy. In N. J. Lass (Ed.), *Speech and language: Advances in basic research and practice* (Vol. X). New York: Academic Press.

Kuhl, P. (1981). Discrimination of speech by nonhuman animals: Basic auditory sensitivities conducive to the perception of speech-sound categories. *Journal of the Acoustical Society of America, 70,* 340–349.

Kuhl, P. (1983). Perception of auditory equivalence classes for speech in early infancy. *Infant Behavior and Development, 6,* 263–285.

Kuhl, P. (1986). Theoretical contributions of tests on animals to the special-mechanisms debate in speech. *Experimental Biology, 45,* 233–265.

Kuhl, P. (1987). Perception of speech and sound in early infancy. In P. Salapatek & L. Cohen (Eds.), *Handbook of Infant Perception* (Vol. 2, pp. 275–382). New York: Academic Press.

Kuhl, P., & Miller, J., (1975). Speech perception by the chinchilla: Voiced-voiceless distinction in alveolar plosive consonants. *Science, 190,* 69-72.

Kuhl, P., & Miller, J. (1978). Speech perception by the chinchilla: Identification functions for synthetic VOT stimuli. *Journal of the Acoustical Society of America, 63,* 905–917.

Kuhl, P., Williams, K., Lacerda, F., Stevens, K., & Lindblom, B. (1992). Linguistic experience alters phonetic perception in infants by 6 months of age. *Science, 255,* 1003–1010.

Ladefoged, P. (1975). *A Course in Phonetics.* New York: Harcourt Brace Jovanovich.

Ladefoged, P., DeClerk, J., Lindau, M., & Papcun, G. (1972). An auditory motor theory of speech production. *UCLA Phonetics Laboratory, Working Papers in Phonetics, 22,* 48–76.

Leonard, L., McGregor, K., & Allen, G. (1992). Grammatical morphology and speech perception in children with Specific Language Impairment. *Journal of Speech and Hearing Research, 35*, 1076–1085.

Liberman, A., Cooper, F., Shankweiler, D., & Studdert-Kennedy, M. (1967). Perception of the speech code. *Psychological Review, 74*, 431–461.

Liberman, A., & Mattingly, I. (1985).The motor theory of speech perception revised. *Cognition, 21*, 1–36.

Lieberman, P. (1975). *On the Origins of Language: An Introduction to the Evolution of Human Speech*. New York: Macmillan.

Lieberman, P. (1984). *The Biology and Evolution of Language*. Cambridge, MA: Harvard University Press.

Lieberman, P., & Blumstein, S. (1988). *Speech Acoustics, Physiology and Perception*. London: Cambridge University Press.

Lisker, L., & Abramson, A. (1964). A cross-language study of voicing in initial stops: Acoustical measurements. *Word, 20*, 384–422.

Lisker, L., & Abramson, A. (1967). Some effects of context on voice onset time in English stops. *Language and Speech, 10*, 1–28.

Marslen-Wilson, W. (1980). Speech understanding as a psychological process. In J. Simon (Ed.), *Spoken Language Generation and Understanding*. New York: Reidel Publishing.

Marslen-Wilson, W., & Welsh, A. (1978). Processing interactions and lexical access during word recognition in continuous speech. *Cognitive Psychology, 10*, 29–63.

McClelland, J., Rumelhart, D., and the PDP Research Group. (1986). *Parallel Distributed Processing: Explorations in the Microstructure of Cognition Volume 2: Psychological and Biological Models*. Cambridge, MA: MIT Press.

McGurk, H., & MacDonald, J. (1976). Hearing lips and seeing voices. *Nature, 264*, 746–748.

Mehler, J. (1985). Language-related dispositions in early infancy. In J. Mehler & R. Fox (Eds.), *Neonate Cognition: Beyond the blooming buzzing confusion*. Hillsdale, NJ: Erlbaum.

Miller, G., & Nicely, P. (1955). An analysis of perceptual confusions among some English consonants. *Journal of the Acoustical Society of America, 27*(2), 338–352.

Neary, T. (1976). *Phonetic Features for Vowels*. Bloomington, IN: Indiana University Linguistics Club.

Owens, E., Talbott, C., & Schubert, E. (1968). Vowel discrimination of hearing-impaired listeners. *Journal of Speech and Hearing Research, 11*, 648–655.

Peretz, I., Morais, J., & Bertelson, P. (1987). Shifting ear differences in melody recognition through strategy inducement. *Brain and Cognition, 6*, 202–215.

Pisoni, D. (1978). Speech perception. In W. Estes (Ed.), *Handbook of Learning and Cognitive Processes* (Vol. 6.). Hillsdale, NJ: Erlbaum.

Polka, L., & Werker, J. (1994). Developmental changes in the perception of non-native vowel contrasts. *Journal of Experimental Psychology: Human Perception & Performance, 20,* 421–435.

Repp, B. (1988). Acoustic properties and perception of stop consonant release transients. *Journal of the Acoustical Society of America. 85*(1), 379–396.

Rumelhart, D., McClelland, J., and the PDP Research Group. (1986). *Parallel Distributed Processing: Explorations in the Microstructure of Cognition Volume 1: Foundations.* Cambridge, MA: MIT Press.

Ryalls, J. (1986). Synesthesia: A principle for the relationship between the primary colors and the cardinal vowels. *Semiotica, 58,* 107–121.

Ryalls, J. (1987a). Vowel perception in aphasia. *Clinical Linguistics & Phonetics, 1*(1), 91–95.

Ryalls, J. (1987b). Vowel production in aphasia: Towards an account of the consonant-vowel dissociation. In J. Ryalls (Ed.), *Phonetic Approaches to Speech Production in Aphasia and Related Disorders* (Chapter 2). Boston, MA: College-Hill Press.

Ryalls, J., Baum, S., & Larouche, A. (1991). Spectral characteristics for place of articulation in the speech of young normal, moderately and profoundly hearing-impaired French Canadians. *Clinical Linguistics and Phonetics, 5*(2), 165–179.

Samuel, A. (1981). Phonemic restoration: Insights from a new methodology. *Journal of Experimental Psychology: General, 110*(4), 474–494.

Shankweiler, D., & Studdert-Kennedy, M. (1967). Identification of consonants and vowels presented to left and right ears. *Quarterly Journal of Experimental Psychology, 19,* 59–63.

Shinn, P., & Blumstein, S. (1983). Phonetic disintegration in aphasia: Acoustic analysis of spectral characteristics for place of articulation. *Brain and Language, 20,* 90–114.

Sidtis, J. (1982). Predicting brain organization from dichotic listening performance: Cortical and subcortical functional asymmetries contribute to perceptual asymmetries. *Brain and Language, 17,* 287–300.

Singh, S., & Singh, K. (1982). *Phonetics: Principles and Practices* (2nd Edition). Austin, TX: Pro-Ed.

Sinott, J., Beecher, M., Moody, D., & Stebbins, W. (1976). Speech sound discrimination by monkeys and humans. *Journal of the Acoustical Society of America, 60,* 687–695.

Speaks, C. (1992). *Introduction to Sound: Acoustics for the Hearing and Speech Sciences.* San Diego, CA: Singular.

Stevens, K., & Blumstein, S. (1978). Invariant cues for place of articulation in stop consonants. *Journal of the Acoustical Society of America, 64,* 1358–1368.

Stevens, K., & Blumstein, S. (1981). The search for invariant acoustic correlates of phonetic features. In P. Eimas & J. Miller (Eds.),

Perspectives on the Study of Speech (pp. 1–38). Hillsdale, NJ: Erlbaum.

Stevens, K., & Halle, M. (1967). Remarks on analysis-by-synthesis and distinctive features. In W. Wathen-Dunn (Ed.), *Models for the Perception of Speech and Visual Form.* Cambridge, MA: MIT Press.

Strange, W. (1986). Speech input and the development of speech perception. In J. Kavanaugh (Ed.), *Otitis Media and Child Development.* Parkton, MD: York Press.

Sussman, J. (1993). Perception of formant transition cues to place of articulation in children with language impairments. *Journal of Speech and Hearing Research, 36*, 1286–1299.

Tallal, P., Miller, S., & Fitch, R. (1993). Neurobiological basis of speech: A case for the preeminence of temporal processing. In. P. Tallal, A. Gallaburda, R. Llinas, & C. von Euler (Eds.), *Temporal Processing in the Nervous System* (pp. 27–47). *Annals of the New York Academy of Sciences, 682.*

Verbrugge, R., Strange, W., Shankweiler, D., & Erdman, T. (1976). What information enables a listener to map a talker's vowel space? *Journal of the Acoustical Society of America, 60*, 198–212.

Warren, R. (1970). Perceptual restoration of missing speech sounds. *Science, 167*, 392–393.

Waters, R., & Wilson, W.A. Jr. (1976). Speech perception by rhesus monkeys: The voicing distinction in synthesized labial and velar stop consonants. *Perception and Psychophysics, 19*, 285–289.

Werker, J. (1989). Becoming a native listener. *American Scientist, 77*, 55–59.

Werker, J., & Pegg, J. (1992). Infant speech perception and phonological acquisition. In C. Ferguson, L. Menn, & C. Stoel-Gammon (Eds.), *Phonological Development: Models, Research and Implications.* Parkton, MD: York Press.

Werker, J., & Polka, L. (1993). Developmental changes in speech perception: New challenges and new directions. *Journal of Phonetics, 21*, 83–101.

Werker, J. & Tess., R. (1984). Cross-language speech perception: Evidence for perceptual reorganization during the first year of life. *Infant Behavior and Development, 7*, 49–63.

Wernicke, C. (1874). *Der aphasische Symptomenkomplex.* Breslau, Germany: Cohn & Weigert.

Wernicke, C. (1908). The symptomcomplex of aphasia. In A. Church (Ed.), *Modern Clinical Medecine* (pp. 265–324). New York: Appleton.

Whitfield, J., & Evans, E. (1965). Responses of auditory cortical neurons to stimuli of changing frequency. *Journal of Neurophysiology, 28*, 655–672.

Index